Jason Padgett had struggled as a student and has spent his professional life working at his father's shop, Planet Futon. Following a mugging outside a bar in 2002 he became agoraphobic and during that time at home he developed an unprecedented passion for learning. A chance encounter in a mall with a university physicist encouraged him to return to college where his genius is discovered, particularly his unique ability to hand draw mathematical fractals. He has Acquired Savant Syndrome and synesthesia and is believed to be unique.

Maureen Seaberg is a science journalist, and as a synesthete herself focuses on writing about synesthesia. She met Jason as a result of Google alert on the subject and introduced him to the neuroscientist that diagnosed his condition.

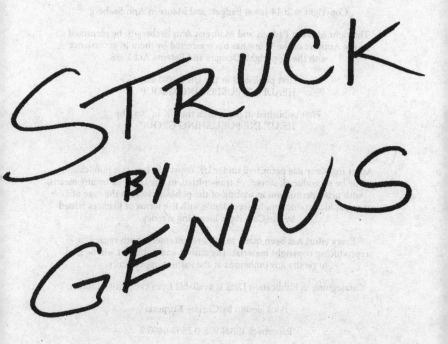

STRUCK BY GENIUS

JASON PADGETT

AND MAUREEN SEABERG

headline

The right of Jason Padgett and Maureen Ann Seaberg to be identified
as the Authors of the Work has been asserted by them in accordance
with the Copyright, Designs and Patents Act 1988.

First published in the UK in 2014 by
HEADLINE PUBLISHING GROUP

First published in paperback the UK in 2015 by
HEADLINE PUBLISHING GROUP

1

Cataloguing in Publication Data is available from the British Library

Book design by Chrissy Kurpeski

Paperback ISBN 978 0 7553 6460 2

Typeset in Warnock Pro
Printed and bound in the UK by Clays Ltd, St Ives plc

All images courtesy of the author, with the following exceptions: 2s and
5s, p. 68, courtesy of V. S. Ramachandran; mathematical equation, p. 110,
courtesy of Naomi Gibbs; Klüver's Form Constants, p. 157, copyright © 2002,
Massachusetts Institute of Technology, from "What Geometric Visual
Hallucinations Tell Us about the Visual Cortex," by Paul C. Bressloff,
Jack D. Cowan, Martin Golubtisky, Peter J. Thomas, and Matthew C. Wiener.

MIX
Paper from
responsible sources
FSC® C104740

Headline's policy is to use papers that are natural, renewable and recyclable
products and made from wood grown in well-managed forests and other
controlled sources. The logging and manufacturing processes are expected to
conform to the environmental regulations of the country of origin.

HEADLINE PUBLISHING GROUP
An Hachette UK Company
338 Euston Road
London NW1 3BH

www.headline.co.uk
www.hachette.co.uk

Contents

Contents

A Note from Maureen

I'VE NEVER MET anyone like Jason Padgett, yet he reminds me of my brother, my neighbor, my mailman, and the guy behind the deli counter up the street. He's just a likable, salt-of-the-earth, sweet fellow wrapped up in the most extraordinary of circumstances, almost as though he woke up one morning and swallowed the sun.

I had an immediate and visceral reaction to his story when I first stumbled upon it, and during our initial e-mail exchanges, he patiently responded to my incredulous reactions (yes, he'd suffered a traumatic brain injury during a mugging, and no, he'd never been able to draw like that before) and gave me the specifics of his experience, which dropped my jaw at every turn. But it was really the way he opened up to me (I was a complete stranger, after all), the warmth and passion and optimism he brought to even the lowest points of his story, that convinced me of his star quality. Two weeks later, when we finally met in person, my fate was sealed.

It was clear that he'd completely rebounded from his severe agoraphobia and rediscovered the joy of conversation, and whether he was speaking to the cashier who sold us lunch that afternoon or the neuroscientists he mingled with months later — or me, for that matter — he was charming, humble, and, most of all, inspiring. What happened to Jason couldn't have happened to a kinder, more genuine, or more innocent person, and the fact that he survived years of insecurity, paranoia, and fear and found his way back to being as magnetic as ever, only with a truer sense of purpose, never ceases to give me hope. When you meet Jason, talk to him on the phone, or see him onstage, it takes only a few seconds to see the innate good in him that preceded and outlasted his injury, and it takes only a few seconds to start seeing the world with as much wonder as he does.

When Jason agreed with me that his story should be told, he admitted that he could no longer write particularly well, and he has found that his desire to read about subjects that don't relate to math is greatly diminished. He was never much of an English student even before his assault, and after it, those skills he had seemed to decline, an unfortunate side effect of his brain injury. (I should point out that he handles this and myriad other tradeoffs with tremendous grace.) I, however, was a writer eager for such a profound story. I've had synesthesia — a neurological phenomenon causing the blending of senses — ever since I was a child, but I never encountered anything like Jason's mathematical, empirical synesthesia. We had some of each other's puzzle pieces, so we decided to team up. It is Jason's voice you will hear in the pages that follow, as we tell his story together.

Along this journey, Jason and I have logged thousands of miles, meeting in New York, Sweden, Wisconsin, and Washington. We've spent hundreds of hours on the telephone and writing e-mail. We've pondered the cosmos and consciousness and life itself in the kind of conversation usually reserved for late nights in college residence halls. We've laughed a lot and we've cried together too. I have been humbled and inspired a thousand times over. I thank his wife, Elena, and his daughter, Megan, for sharing this incredible human being with me and for giving me the chance to share his story with you.

Struck by Genius

CHAPTER ONE

Jason 2.0

I F YOU COULD see the world through my eyes, you would know how perfect it is, how much order runs through it, and how much structure is hidden in its tiniest parts. We're so often victims of things — I see the violence too, the disease, the poverty stretching far and wide — but the universe itself and everything we can touch and all that we are is made of the most beautiful geometric patterns imaginable. I know because they're right in front of me. Because of a traumatic brain injury, the result of a brutal physical attack, I've been able to see these patterns for over a decade. This change in my perception was really a change in my brain function, the result of the injury and the extraordinary and mostly positive way my brain healed. All of a sudden, the patterns were just . . . *there*, and I realize now that my injury was a rare gift. I'm lucky to have survived, but for me, the real miracle — what really saved me — was being introduced to and almost overwhelmed by the mathematical grace of the universe.

There's a park in my town of Tacoma, Washington, that I like to walk through in the mornings before work. I see the trees that line its path as anyone would, the branches and the bark, but I see a geometrical blueprint laid on top of them too. I see triangular patterns emerging from the leaves, reminding me of the Pythagorean theorem, as if it's unfolding in the air, proving to me over and over again what the ancient Greek philosopher and mathematician Pythagoras deduced thousands of years ago: the sum of the squares of the legs of a right triangle (a triangle in which one angle is a right angle, or 90 degrees) equals the square of its hypotenuse. I don't need a calculator to know that the simple formula most of us learned in school — $a^2 + b^2 = c^2$ — is true; I can see it instantly in the trees all around me. To me, a tree is more than its geometry, but geometry is also far more than most people realize. I think it's everything.

I remember reading that Galileo Galilei, the Italian astronomer, mathematician, and physicist (and one of my heroes), said that we cannot understand the universe until we have learned its language. He said, "It is written in the language of mathematics, and its characters are triangles, circles, and other geometric figures, without which it is humanly impossible to understand a single word of it."

This rings true for me. I see this hidden language of the world before my eyes.

Doctors tell me that nothing in my brain was newly created or added when I was injured. Rather, innate but dormant skills were released. This theory comes from psychiatrist Darold Treffert, who is considered the world's leading authority on savants and acquired savants. He treated the late Kim Peek (the inspiration for the savant character in the movie *Rain Man*), a megasavant who memorized twelve thousand books, including the Bible and the Book of Mormon, but who had so many physical challenges that he had to rely on his father for his most basic needs. When I met with Dr. Treffert in his hometown of Fond du Lac, Wisconsin, he told me that these innate skills are, in his words, "factory-installed software" or "genetic" memory. After interviewing me in his office and in his home, he declared that my acquired synesthesia and savant syndrome was self-evident, and he also suggested that all of us have extraordinary skills just beneath the surface, much as birds innately know how to fly in a V-formation and fish know how to swim in a school. Why the brain suppresses these remarkable abilities is still a mystery, but sometimes, when the brain is diseased or damaged, it relents and unleashes the inner genius. This isn't just my story. It's the story of the potential secreted away in all of us.

The first thing I do every morning is make my way to the bathroom, turn on the faucet, and let the sink fill up. I watch the water flow and wonder why it doesn't sound like the strumming of tightly wound strings. The structure of flowing water vibrates in a specific geometric form and frequency to me, and if it were to freeze midstream, I'd see a web, but one made up of tiny crystals rather than spider's silk. If I could hear it after it froze, it would sound like tinkling glass shards falling into the basin. I like to start my days with water. It may slip through my fingers, but it is a constant comfort.

I look at myself in the mirror and make sure my hair's not getting too long. I like it cropped close now. I grab my toothbrush and count how many times I run it through the water while brushing my teeth. It has to be exactly sixteen times. I don't know why I chose that number, but it's fixed in my mind like my street address or my zip code. I try not to worry about it too much and stare back at the intriguing water webs, working to memorize all of the angles so that I can draw a picture of the image later. I'll probably spend hours with a pencil and ruler later on, capturing on paper every inch of the razor-sharp symmetry.

Next, I walk into the living room and throw back the drapes. If it's a clear day, I'm in for a real show. The sun comes shining through the leaves of the trees like a million little lights, as if the leaves are blades and they cut the sun up into a million diamonds. Then the rays fan out between the leaves, falling over them like an illuminated net. Watching this, I always think of the famous double-slit experiment, in which light behaves like a particle and a wave at the same time. My friends tell me that to them, it's just the sun shining through the trees. I can barely remember a time when I saw the world the way most everyone else does.

On an overcast or stormy day, I pay more attention to the branches swaying in the wind. The movements are choppy and discrete, like a series of frames of a film, with black lines separating each image. At first, I got dizzy when this happened, and I had to grab the back of a chair or lean against a wall. Now I'm used to it, though I still have moments of vertigo.

Next I move on to the kitchen and put on some coffee. It's one of my routines, but it thrills me every single time I watch the cream being stirred into the brew. That perfect spiral is an important shape to me. It's a fractal — a repetitive geometric form found everywhere in nature, from the shell of a nautilus up to the Milky Way galaxy. Suddenly it's not just my morning cup of joe — awesome as the coffee in the Pacific Northwest is — it's geometry speaking to me again. And I never get tired of it.

I sit down at the kitchen table and add to whatever sketch I'm working on; lately, I've been drawing the coffee-and-cream spiral. I'm a real perfectionist and I can stay in my seat for hours and draw; usually, I do this until I have to leave for work. When it's finally time to go, I put on my "uniform" — a button-down shirt and jeans. I like to look professional but I'm not really one to wear a suit and I often have to lift heavy things or repair stuff at work. I make sure I close the door behind me carefully. I always have to check and double-check and triple-check the locks. Then I can go.

I used to drive my wife, Elena, to school in the morning. I did it partly because I like spending as much time as possible with her, but it was also a matter of her safety. Until very recently, we lived in a not-so-friendly part of Tacoma called Hilltop. Our house was next door to a soup kitchen, and while I was sympathetic to its patrons, a few of the folks were tough characters. Sometimes it was like running a gauntlet in the alley beside our house just to get to our car. I could handle it, but if anyone ever hurt Elena, I don't know what I'd do. Some of the homeless people hung out on our porch waiting for the soup kitchen to open. One time I tripped over a man sleeping at the foot of our front door. He just moaned and didn't move an inch.

Owing to the nearby jail, our street was filled with storefront offices that housed bail bondsmen and defense lawyers, and the foot traffic was made up of people who required their services. Many of them were gang members. A lot of the crimes they were accused of stemmed from the crack and methamphetamine epidemics in Washington State. During the twelve years I lived there, I came to recognize a lot of the characters; they showed up again and again — repeat offenders, I guess. Even the name of the local sandwich place was inspired by the atmosphere: the 911 Deli. Lunch emergencies were the least of my neighborhood's problems.

But the location was convenient for me and Elena because we both attended nearby colleges. Elena was studying business, and I'd returned to school to learn all I could about math and physics. I'd dropped out years before my injury due to poor grades and the fact that school just didn't interest me. I made it through only half of my sophomore year of college. I had to drop out again a few years ago to take care of my health and the family business, but I recently re-enrolled. My instructors say I have an incredible and inexplicable grasp of theory, considering that I've never studied these subjects formally before, but I still need to learn the basics. Although it's easy for me to understand the mathematical nature of the universe now, I don't have the background to express it verbally. But I'm really happy to be in school. For the first time in my life, I'm taking my education seriously.

During my morning drives, which now start at Browns Point, I sing along to the radio and do my best to concentrate on the traffic, but there's a lot competing for my attention. I'm constantly watching the light play off cars, including the hood of my own, and it seems to signal to me something about the relative speeds of vehicles on the road. The length of the light between the cars I see in stop-action frames is a short filament; when things move faster, this light stream is longer. I found out in school that this image I see could be a textbook description of accepted theories on derivatives of position and velocity that lead to acceleration in physics. I find it's more reliable to react to these visuals than to people's brake lights. The shape of the sky itself as I look out my windshield can be a distraction too. Its half-dome curvature reminds me of pi, the irrational number that represents the circumference of a circle divided by its diameter. Most of us have seen pi written as 3.14 or 3.14159, but the digits actually never end. Pi goes on into infinity and never repeats, which is why it's called an irrational number and also why it's so fascinating to me. I draw pi constantly as a circle subdivided by triangles, and I've gotten so that I can fit 720 triangles into the circle. I'd put more in there but that's the highest number I can produce before the width of the pencil lead causes the lines to run together.

When I drive past the city's harbor — Commencement Bay — I'm always on the lookout for rainbows. The stormy conditions of Washington State turn the sky over this body of water — full of frolicking seals and the occasional orca — into a real rainbow factory in spite of the industrial smokestacks spewing smog into the air overhead. Each time I see one I'm reminded of their geometry. To me, they are a reflection of pi. I'm apt to pull over the car and text people when I see an exceptional one: *Double bow! Three o'clock!*

My first stop after passing the harbor is often the office of the doctor or the physical therapist to deal with chronic pain from old injuries. Both offices tend to be busy, and I usually have to wait, but I have no problem keeping myself occupied. Downtime gives me the opportunity to think.

While other patients reach for the dog-eared magazines, I imagine myself shrinking down to a microscopic level, no larger than a bacterium. My perspective shifts until I can no longer see the ceiling above me, and the end table in the corner of the room sprawls out like a giant, unexplored plain. I begin taking microscopic steps, and I come upon a spot on the table where a fellow patient's filling out her paperwork, pressing her ballpoint pen into the medical form's surface. After she finishes and moves the paper aside, I find myself lost in the huge crater: the indent in the wood formed when she dotted an *i*. Like an explorer, I hike its entirety, traversing the valley in half an hour or so and looking at the grains of the wood as if I were in the middle of a gargantuan forest. I climb to the surface and look across the expanse of the indents left from the other letters and numbers she wrote. They spread out before me like the mysterious Nazca lines of Peru and I forget for a moment how they were made and puzzle over them. When the receptionist calls my name, I'm pulled out of the rabbit hole, and I walk into the office thinking that this is my particular theory of relativity. The table looks smooth from a human perspective, but we'd need only to shrink down to a smaller perspective to experience the textures I imagined. Everything is relative to your place in the world. Speaking of which, I'm also a real champ at waiting in line at the bank. I think it's a stroke of luck not to know boredom anymore.

Despite my very rich inner life, like anyone, I have to come back down to earth to deal with the day-to-day business of survival. I make my living at a place called Planet Futon. Seriously. When I get to work, there are usually a dozen fires to put out right away that snap me out of my reverie and into the here and now. It's a family business. My dad owns the furniture factory in Illinois that supplies our three stores in the Tacoma area, and I have managed them for him on and off since 2001, spending most of my time at the flagship store. It's important to have a member of the family in charge, otherwise people might rob you blind. I know because I took a little time off recently, and it wasn't long before one of the workers was offering customers discounts for using cash, delivering the furniture himself, and then keeping the money. Also, if a piece of furniture is missing a part, the workers tend to poach that part off the brand-new furniture instead of just ordering it, which creates a cascade of problems. The stores support not only my household but also my dad's. Most of the responsibility of making them profitable falls on my shoulders. As grateful as I am for the job, it puts a tremendous amount of pressure on me, and I don't handle stress as well as I used to. In the old days, I met it head-on, but now I avoid any and all confrontations. This new personality trait is something my doctors consider a tradeoff, a drawback that comes with my new abilities.

As hard as it is to manage employees and keep the fleet of delivery trucks humming, I enjoy my interactions with our customers. Some salespeople talk to shoppers about the weather or last night's game to break the ice, and that's fine. I used to do the same thing. But now I talk to them about geometry and physics. You'd be surprised how positively people respond — even people who didn't think they cared a whit about either topic. The trick is to make it relevant. It's as easy as describing the mechanism of the fulcrum that opens a futon; I do that, and we're off.

I'm forty-three as of this writing. This makes me really happy because 43 is a prime number, divisible by only itself and 1. The number 43 lives at a specific point in a sphere in my mind's eye, as do all the other primes. I've drawn images of this sphere, which is consistent for me whenever I think of primes and the patterns among them. I feel such a reverence for these numbers that I recite them like a mantra when I need good luck or when I need to keep bad luck away. It's as if the primes are so rare and so special that they're imbued with an extraordinary power, and they act like sentinels in my mind. When I'm napping on the sofa, my daughter, Megan, sometimes wakes me up because I'm reciting prime numbers in my sleep.

But primes aren't the only numbers I associate with shapes. Simply dialing a friend's phone number can send up a plume of images. Numbers appear to me as a series of cubes. They are linear — three cubes across for the number 3, four across for 4 — unless the numbers are part of an equation or they're being plotted on a graph, in which case the cubes move around to reflect what's happening to the numbers. An equation can result in a huge, prismatic net right before my eyes. The shapes are always consistent with the specific stimulus. Numbers are an obsession, and I'm incapable of turning the fixation off. I can't climb stairs without counting them, and I can't eat without counting how many times I've chewed each bite. I never chew gum for this reason. With every number I count off, the fresh, simple prime numbers and all the other never-ending numbers spiral into their own shapes.

All these visions — and every shape I encounter out in the world — correlate with fractals, the elemental geometric building blocks found in nature. Snowflakes, lightning bolts, and coastlines are all fractals, meaning their subsections repeat the same patterns as their wholes. Coastlines are particularly intriguing to me because their overall measurements actually change depending on the scale one uses. For me, this underscores how understanding fractals can shed light on comprehending the nature of other things. For example, I have always wanted to know where humans come from. Now, with one quick glance at human anatomy, I see clearly that veins, arteries, and even the strands of DNA are fractals too. The human body seems to reflect the very structure of creation. The structures within the body reflect the never-ending repeating patterns found throughout the universe. The first time I noticed this, it struck me: everything and everyone is a reflection of this repeating structure.

I walk around in a near-constant state of inspiration with a great hunger for knowledge, and I read everything I can about math and physics, often developing my own theories along the way. I was even contacted by a Toronto financial firm that was interested in applying my fractal geometry to the stock market. I haven't begun working with them yet, but I love the idea that my wild visions could have an application in the real world.

It's especially important for me to keep drawing my geometry, because that's how I'm able to share exactly what's going on in my mind, and I think I'd go crazy if I didn't have a way to express what I see. By turning my view of the world into drawings, I've found a way to explain my universe to other people.

My quest to understand and come to terms with the new me has spanned more than a decade, taking me from years of self-imposed isolation to a high-tech brain-imaging lab halfway across the world, in Helsinki, Finland. Along the way, I've met some of the world's greatest experts on savant syndrome, synesthesia, and brain science. I've learned what my mathematical theories and visions have in common with the work of some of the most brilliant mathematicians in history. I've been introduced to new ways of thinking about the brain, the mind, and even consciousness, and I've discovered why my case may play an instrumental role in the next generation of cutting-edge brain science.

I've spent plenty of time pondering the very fabric of the universe and how we fit into it. And I've concluded that no matter what you go through in life, in the end, there is a symmetry to it all — an order amid the seeming disorder. And if you could see what I see, you'd know that you're an essential part of that order.

If I could draw the world as I see it and show every last person how he or she is enmeshed in this fine and intricate and impossibly beautiful structure, perhaps people would stop getting lost in the hurt of things and be elevated by the wonder of it all. In fact, I know they would. I know, because even though I seem like the most optimistic man this side of the Rocky Mountains, I've been to hell and back.

Jason 1.0

THERE WAS ONCE a time when, apart from tallying my bar tab or cashing my paycheck or counting repetitions when I did curls at the gym, I was blissfully unaware of mathematics. In fact, I was more than unaware; I was math-averse. In school, I was like so many other students: the only questions I had for my math teachers were "When am I going to use that?" and "How does this apply to anything in the real world?" I never made it past prealgebra, much less developed any theories about the geometric underpinnings of the universe.

Back then, nothing I was taught in school seemed relevant. I wasn't motivated and I got terrible grades. I didn't have much of an attention span. I liked to party. I was an adrenaline junkie, always in search of the next fix. Eventually I dropped out of college.

Life was meant to be enjoyed, after all, and there was nothing fun about math or science or academic pursuits of any kind — all of which required sitting still. I was out every night of the week after school or after work. Now, that was fun. My main concerns were where I'd be partying that night, which girls I'd be meeting, and what drinks I'd be drinking. When I lived in Alaska, which I did on and off through my teens and early twenties, that meant meeting Justin, John, Rick, and Alicia at Chilkoot Charlie's ("Where we cheat the other guy and pass the savings on to you!"); Hot Rods, with its lineup of muscle cars on display; or Asia Gardens, for a little (or a lot of) karaoke. When I was in Tacoma, my entourage was Angela, Tina, and Clark, and we'd end up at either Café Arizona or Shogun's after a game of ultimate Frisbee. I was never alone.

My frequent trips to the gym left my biceps bulging; I wore cut-off T-shirts to better display my muscles. My hair was long and heavy with styling products. My favorite outfit to go out in was tight jeans, no shirt, and a leather vest. I wince now when I think of this getup, sort of what a Chippendales dancer would wear. I was just looking for the next good time, sometimes in Alaska and sometimes in Washington State, as I shuttled back and forth between divorced parents.

When I was a teenager I drew up a bucket list—before there were bucket lists—of all the things I wanted to do before I died. When I look back at it now, it actually looks like a list of ways *to* die. And I worked my way through it. Cliff jumping while skiing? Check, a bunch of times. Bungee jumping? At least thirty times, once in Mexico at a shady place that was later shut down for safety violations. Skydiving? Nineteen times. Scuba diving with sharks? Check, in the Bahamas. I broke my hand twice, broke my leg, broke my collarbone, and broke my heel, all for the sake of feeling the rush.

Even before that, I took up martial arts—at the age of twelve— and I earned a brown belt in karate. I loved being physical as much as I loved the thrill I got from the fear of getting hurt. I was prone to boredom; I couldn't even sit still for Saturday-morning cartoons. I avoided feeling bored by keeping myself in constant motion. I was adventurous from the start, and my first memory of experiencing the possibility of danger came from a trip our family went on when I was three years old.

We'd stopped at a little roadside restaurant for something to eat. There were picnic tables out back with a view of Campbell Creek, which at that point was swollen to river proportions from the Alaska spring thaw. I spotted a beach ball floating by, and my parents turned away for just a moment. I stepped into the rushing tributary.

I honestly thought I could walk on water. I knew about puddles, which I'd been able to splash through without harm, so I thought I would just step out and grab the ball. It was a complete shock when I sank into the water and was carried away in the rapids. I couldn't have been more surprised if my foot had gone through asphalt.

My brother was right behind me. With no regard for his own safety, five-year-old John went in after me, and he was also swept away.

I saw my brother by my side in the swirling water as the creek ran into a tunnel under a roadway. Then my head dipped under, and there was darkness. Then daylight — *breathe* — and the sight of long flights of stairs leading up to waterfront homes. River, darkness. Then daylight — *breathe* — and a woman standing on one of those stairways with an armload of groceries. River, darkness. Then daylight — *breathe* — and the sight of all those groceries flying in the air and the woman running toward us. River, darkness. Then daylight — *breathe* — warm bathwater in the lady's home, police officers, worried parents, and John at my side.

My mother and father divorced when I was nine years old. Mom moved with my older brother and me to the pit-stop town of Cantwell, Alaska. She worked as a medevac paramedic for oil and logging companies in the Alaska wilderness, and the town of Cantwell was pretty much just a twelve-room motel, a restaurant, and a gas station. Kids weren't allowed at the motel — not that there were any other kids there — so she rented a small cabin around a bend in the road. We spent our days without running water or electricity. John and I ate our meals together at the restaurant, and we worked in tandem to haul water in a ten-gallon bucket, too heavy for sixty-pound me alone. We played adventurers by gaslight in the cabin and explored the woods, removing surveyors' wooden posts and crafting swords out of them. I knew what it meant to have very little.

I may have been a heat-seeking missile for risk and adventure throughout childhood and young adulthood, but I found myself strongly drawn to people unlike myself. From the start I had a soft spot for shy, quiet people — never more so than when I met a fellow student I'll call Mike after I moved to Washington to be with my dad, when I was ten. Mike was extremely introverted, wore thick Coke-bottle-lens glasses, and was as messy as Pig-Pen in the *Peanuts* comic strip. You just knew he had a story to tell. I was cordial to him even though he was roundly shunned by everyone else, but I didn't really befriend him until my sophomore year of high school, when I was sixteen.

One afternoon I saw him reaching into the cafeteria trash cans when he thought no one was looking, pulling out orange peels and trying to eat the fruit still stuck to them. I couldn't help but stare, and then I noticed the duct tape covering the holes in his jeans. Didn't he have enough money for a patch or a needle and thread? I wondered. Compared to my time in the woods with my mom, I was spoiled with my dad as a teen. My father's furniture business was flourishing, and we lived a comfortable life — we had a grand total of ten cars in the garage and driveway — and I felt pangs of guilt after noticing Mike's situation. Seeing him forage for his lunch reminded me of a time in my life when I barely had the basics myself.

Later that afternoon I asked Mike if he'd like to hang out with me and my best friend at the time, Jeff. He looked completely surprised but said yes, and pretty soon the three of us were thick as thieves.

"Stand up straight, Mike," Jeff would advise him when we were out and about. "Look people in the eye. It's okay." Jeff and I were part of the popular crowd so we even managed to fix him up with a couple of girls.

One day I drove Mike home after we'd all been hanging out. As soon as we entered his house, his mother yelled, "Mike, get out on that bus!" I was sure she didn't mean the derelict yellow school bus I'd noticed in the front yard, but she did. Mike wasn't allowed in the house. His family gave him scraps from the table like a dog. He was embarrassed that I'd seen his home life, and with his head hung low, he explained to me that it was still better than when his biological father was living there.

At that moment I decided to bring Mike home with me. He reminded me of Oliver Twist, a Dickens character I'd played in a local production of *Oliver!* only a few years earlier, when I strongly resembled the actor who played the British orphan in the movie. That day, after hearing Mike's story, my father set up a cot for him in my bedroom, and we washed his clothes and gave him a good meal.

With Mike's new home all ready, I took him back to his house and encouraged him to not only pick up his few possessions but also give his mother and stepfather a piece of his mind. He walked up to his stepfather and screamed "Fuck you!" right into his face. The man went into another room and returned with a pistol. We ran from the house and took off like a shot in my little Datsun (actually the slowest car in the Padgett fleet back then). From that point on, Mike was the third brother in the Padgett household.

On his birthday, we blindfolded him, covered his ears, put him in the car, and took him on a shopping trip. We bought him shoes and all sorts of clothes and had everything gift-wrapped. We went on a total spree with him, which finally ended when we walked him, still blindfolded and earmuffed, into Chuck E. Cheese's. We took off the earmuffs and the blindfold, and he stared at the presents set out on the table for a second, then burst into tears. Jeff and I were trying not to cry ourselves when he told us it was the only birthday of his anyone had ever celebrated.

After we graduated from high school, we lost touch; I was uprooted time and again as my parents went through a series of divorces and remarriages.

Many people who have been shuttled around often in life have trouble making friends. That was never the case with me — my many friends ran the gamut from the shy ones like Mike to those who shared my spirit of adventure. Though I developed a lifelong fear of swimming after the near-drowning incident in Campbell Creek, it didn't stop me from becoming a member of the polar-bear club — a group of people across the nation who are dedicated to braving cold bodies of water — and jumping into the Arctic Ocean years later, when I was working on a northern oil field more than a day's drive from Anchorage. I loved being a "polar bear," and I even saw some of the actual white giants a couple of times during my tenure in the oil fields. Sometimes they looked almost approachable, covering their eyes with their paws or rubbing their noses like in a cartoon. I felt equally at home with people and with nature. I guess you could say I was rugged. I loved the wildness of Alaska and I cultivated a wild streak in myself too.

I remember vividly how the caribou herd on that northern Alaska slope behaved. They reminded me of myself: strong and free and comfortable on the open plain. The large deerlike creatures, thousands of them, were always flicking their ears, whipping their tails, and suddenly bucking or diving into a nearby creek to stave off a swarm of mosquitoes dropping in from above the tundra.

I was twenty years old that first season in the oil fields. I pulled mosquito netting down over my hardhat and taped it to my collar — it looked like a beekeeper's helmet — to avoid the swarm. I'd purchased the netting because my mother, whose new husband had gotten me the job, had warned me that the mosquitoes up north could bite through even blue jeans. It was a rough job, picking up trash in the oil fields on the outskirts of Barrow, near Prudhoe Bay. I was 857 miles north of my hometown of Anchorage and one of only fifty young people chosen out of thousands of applicants for the summer work. And I was lucky to be earning the eleven hundred dollars a week, but the days were long. I had to pull twelve-hour shifts every day for two weeks, then I got two weeks off. The fact that the sun never set made it only a little bit easier.

Swiney, my boss and the biggest roustabout on my crew, considered me a chip off the old hog. He called me Pork Chop, and the nickname stuck. Everyone had a nickname on the oil fields; the two young women who rounded out our group were Cookie Monster and Demon.

"Hey, Pork Chop," Swiney said one day. "Watch this."

Cookie Monster and Demon were out collecting trash about five hundred feet from the Ford pickup truck that was their mobile command center for a dozen hours a day. We all drove trucks specially fitted with two gas tanks, and we had to monitor the fuel levels constantly; the last thing you wanted was to run out of gas somewhere out in the cold, miles from the camp. You had to leave the engine running at all times because if you turned the truck off in the bad weather, it might not start up again. The young women wore beekeepers' helmets too (once they saw mine, they each wanted one, and they paid me ten times more than it cost me to purchase the materials for them), but they had an aversion to carrying the nine-pound air-monitoring devices that would alert them to the presence of hydrogen sulfide gas — known as H_2S around those parts — a lethal byproduct of the drilling that sometimes seeped to the surface of the fields. Swiney, the team leader, had been on their cases about it, but they said it weighed them down too much while they worked. They'd been told repeatedly that at a certain threshold of parts per million, H_2S can shut down human hearts and lungs. Even that information didn't convince them to lug around the monitors.

So that day, Swiney took his own air-monitoring device, put it down by his butt, and farted loudly into the equipment, which immediately set off the machine's warning signals and sent the huge caribou herd galloping. The monitor's alarm and the thundering hooves of thousands of animals were the only sounds in that barren, apocalyptic landscape of scrub and mud.

"H-two-S! H-two-S!" he screamed. The girls dropped the wooden spears that gave us our job description — stick-pickers — and ran for their lives, bumping into each other and repeatedly falling in the mud as they plowed toward the truck to get their gas masks. Swiney and I ran for cover, doubling over with laughter.

Later, a truck full of oil workers came speeding toward our crew. By now, we were used to the crass and randy men who made up the village of five thousand employees. They hung out the window of the truck and whistled and made rude gestures at the women and then threw an open bag of garbage at our feet.

"Job security!" screamed one of the men as they sped away. The oil workers faced serious danger every day, and they resented the fact that we did much safer work but earned nearly as much as they did, and all because each of us had a dad or an uncle or a family friend who was an industry executive and who threw a little nepotism our way. Stick-pickers like us seldom reported the abuse; we knew life would be even worse in that frontier town if we did. We simply leaned over, picked up the trash, and got back to work.

I had a girlfriend named Melissa at the time; she worked on a different crew, and we broke camp rules and trysted together in our off-hours in the barracks where we lived for the season. We hung thick blankets over the windows to block out the midnight sun. Melissa was very pretty and very smart, but we were young and the last thing I wanted was to get too serious.

One day it was particularly cold out on the tundra and I knew Melissa's parka wouldn't be warm enough for her shift, so I lent her my warmest, thickest coat. Both of our crews were sent to clean the field around the landing strip, where a cargo plane had just set down. My group was alongside the plane, parallel to it; Melissa, sitting in her crew's pickup truck, was directly behind the jet. Out of the blue, only minutes after the plane's engine had shut down, it started back up. I turned immediately to Melissa's crew and started jumping and waving for them to get out of the way, but it was too late. I saw the young Eskimo man she worked with go hurtling through the air in the jet wash. I began to run toward them, avoiding the exhaust stream.

When I got to the truck, Melissa was inside and all the windows on the vehicle were blown out. The jacket I'd lent her was pierced everywhere by shards of glass, but the lining was so thick that the glass hadn't cut all the way through, and she'd been wearing her helmet the whole time. I was so relieved she was all right, and I realized how much I really did care for her. Her coworker had only minor injuries, but he could easily have been killed. It was always scary in the oil fields, and always dangerous, but although I hate to admit it, it was also thrilling, all of it.

Somehow we all managed to survive that work assignment and we made it back home to civilization.

When I was in Anchorage, my friend Rick Cordova was my go-to pal for good times. Tall, dark, and handsome, he was popular with the ladies and was always upsetting one jealous boyfriend or another. Sometimes it was just because he showed up to a bar looking really good. He hadn't done anything at all — *yet*. Once we were walking in the mall and some guy with a beef started to run toward him, his arm pulled back to deliver a punch. I yelled, "Duck!" Rick hit the deck, and the guy missed. We were a good team.

When I married Melissa, Rick traveled all the way to our wedding in Montana. Despite Melissa and I not wanting to get too serious, she'd gotten pregnant back in Alaska. One day, right after we found out, I ran into her uncle. He was an oil executive who worked up on the slope. "I know you'll do the right thing," he said sternly. So I did. I proposed.

I'd been incredibly nervous and uncertain about marriage and family at first, but a couple of months before the baby was due, I started to become excited — I wanted to be a father. This made it especially devastating when Jason Padgett Jr. was born premature and lived only a couple of days. He died in my arms as I rocked him back and forth in a chair in a corner of the hospital room. Melissa and I just stood there like zombies during the funeral. He was the only thing that had kept us together, but neither of us realized how much we had wanted him until tragedy struck. Melissa and I clung to each other for another year, then we divorced. I think of her often and of the little boy who bore my name.

If Jason Jr. had lived, I might have settled down and become a real family man. Who knows? Fate had dealt me a different hand and I went right on back to my partying ways. It was just who I was. That's not to say I never had a quiet moment of introspection or that I was totally shallow in those years. There were times in my early life when I took responsibility for myself, and for others too. Still, the majority of my younger years are a blur. I was spinning like a top in pursuit of stimulation. I had to find excitement outside my own mind, as I had very little inner life, and the inner life I did have wasn't anything I wanted to dwell on. As I mentioned, my parents each went through a string of divorces and remarriages, and my brother, John, became increasingly troubled and estranged from the rest of us as he grew older.

Despite my outward happy-go-lucky, party-guy persona, there was an undercurrent of seediness in the club life I lived, from the drama of the promiscuity to the violence of the alcohol-fueled fights. Behavior that was cute or at least expected when I was in my twenties — boys will be boys, after all — became a little sad when I was in my thirties, as I kept to the same habits while most everyone else was settling down.

By that point I'd had another child, a beautiful daughter named Megan, with one of my girlfriends, Michelle. I was overjoyed when she was born healthy, and I loved her completely, but marrying her mother wasn't something that appealed to me, and it didn't appeal to Michelle either. For a while, we rented on the same floor in the same apartment building so that Megan could just run between our homes and have us both near. But having a daughter didn't change my partying ways. As long as I kept moving, kept drinking, kept hooking up and laughing, I didn't have to face anything inside that might be troubling me.

I'd fallen short of everyone's early expectations for my future. I'd scored very high on an IQ test administered in elementary school, and my father swore from that day forward that I was a genius, but subsequent tests I took online were not as promising, and I gave up on my mind and its potential and just lived for the thrills of adrenaline rushes and good parties. In the battle between mind and body, my physicality had won. In my early twenties, I'd decided I would run my father's furniture stores by day and party every night. I thought I would go on that way forever.

CHAPTER THREE

Subtraction

AT AGE THIRTY-ONE, I guess I was pretty aimless, but it didn't feel like that to me at the time. I was having fun, bouncing from one night out to the next. I rarely had a serious thought in my head. My only goal was to live with joyful abandon 24-7. And in all honesty, I was really happy.

When my friend Angela called from a karaoke bar on a September night in 2002, I was especially excited to join the party. I knew at least twenty karaoke selections by heart; I didn't even have to look at the subtitles on the prompter. My top two songs were "Close My Eyes Forever," by Ozzy Osbourne and Lita Ford, and "Takin' Care of Business," by Bachman-Turner Overdrive. I was a good singer, and I loved the reaction I got from the crowds when I took the stage. Sometimes they really, truly cheered for me. I tried not to let this go to my head when I performed, but I used to squint and imagine I was in a stadium filled with a hundred thousand people. So I was looking forward to another karaoke night with friends.

But first I had to get ready.

I put my Charlie Daniels Band CD in my stereo and began bopping around the house playing air fiddle to "The Devil Went Down to Georgia." I always did a warm-up before going out, to get the adrenaline flowing. I knew the words to this song by heart, but that night I came up with new lyrics based on the line in the original hit song where the hero, Johnny, tells the devil, "Come on back if you ever want to try again." I guess I was always one to tempt fate. It was a thrilling scenario: a rematch with the Prince of Darkness.

I sang:

It had been several years since these two had first met
And unbeknownst to Johnny, the contest wasn't over yet . . .

When the devil spotted Johnny basking in the sun
Enjoying all that wealth from the golden fiddle he had won . . .

The devil said to Johnny, "This time I'll let you start the show,"
But it took Johnny twenty minutes to find his fiddle and his bow.

What if the devil found Johnny years later, bloated and lazy after having won the golden fiddle in the first competition, and challenged him to try again? What if Johnny was foolish enough to gamble his soul one more time? Still dancing, I grabbed a pen and paper, and in the lyrics I found flowing out of me, the devil jumped up on the trunk of Johnny's new Mercedes-Benz and proceeded to annihilate him in competitive fiddling. Johnny lost the challenge, and his children looked on in horror as he fell to the ground and the devil collected his soul in a leather pouch. This was a really good sequel, I decided.

I sang my new version of the song in the shower, and then I began the business of fixing my hair. My hair was long—okay, it was an actual mullet—and I needed a special brush and plenty of mousse and gel and just the right flick of the wrist while blow-drying to get my bangs the way I wanted them. It was brisk weather outside so I piled on the hairspray and dressed in a long-sleeved shirt and my black leather jacket.

It was Friday the thirteenth, but I wasn't superstitious. The bar was in a sketchy part of town, but I'd never had a problem before and I wasn't one to pass up a night out. I made my way upstairs to the second floor of the Mexican restaurant where the bar was located, turned left, and found Angela and her date sitting near the stage. The lighting was dim except for some Christmas-tree lights, a standard bar trick to make everyone look more attractive. How many times had I stayed at a bar until closing and then discovered, when the bright lights were turned on, that the young woman I'd been kissing wasn't nearly as cute as I'd thought? And perhaps under fluorescent lights, I wasn't her ideal man either.

There wasn't much of a crowd, and the place wasn't exactly rocking like a lot of other bars I went to. For me, a good bar was a spot where people were packed in like sardines, the music was so loud you could feel it thumping in your chest, and eight or nine bouncers had to pull guys off one another a few times a night. That kind of place wasn't always safe, but I loved the energy—I loved rough-and-tumble good times. There were no bouncers at the karaoke bar that night, and even if there had been, they wouldn't have had anything to do. It was that quiet.

I made my way to Angela's table, and people handed the DJ, a cross-dressing man named Cat with long fingernails and eye makeup, slips of paper with their song choices. I knew the song I wanted to do; in fact, I even knew its number in the catalog: 34-A-7. I didn't even have to look it up. First up was a newly divorced man who sang Jerry Reed's "She Got the Goldmine (I Got the Shaft)." We all clapped along with him and cheered as he screamed out the bitter lyrics. He definitely felt better by the end of the performance. Angela got her chance a few songs after that and did a perfect "Whatever Lola Wants" from *Damn Yankees*, which was her signature song, and a little while later, I stood at the microphone serenading the crowd of about thirty people with a Jon Bon Jovi song.

Shot down in a blaze of glory
Take me now, but know the truth.

I used the stage well, walking back and forth with a cowboy gait, and when the tune ended, I took a bow to enthusiastic applause. A couple of people shook my hand and declared it awesome. That made me happy. I was lucky enough to get good reactions after most of my performances. The only time I was ever heckled was when I attempted "The Humpty Dance," by Digital Underground, and people started yelling, "White boy!"

I walked to the bar and ordered a Coke, and the tall, brunette bartender's eyes lingered a second too long on my full wallet, but it didn't quite register. I was carrying only a couple hundred dollars, but I had it in small bills so it must have seemed like a real bankroll. I tipped her two dollars and she smiled, then I downed the soda and motioned for my friends to start packing up so I could give them a ride home. They were a little drunk, and half the reason Angela had called me was so that I could play the designated driver, something we often did for each other. My parents had worked hard to teach me about the dangers of drinking and driving. One night I walked eleven miles home in several feet of Alaska snow rather than take the wheel.

Angela and her date and I made our way down the stairs, followed by two other patrons whom I'd seen sitting in the corner of the bar with their backs to the wall.

I was just ten steps out the front door when a blow struck my head just behind my right ear. There was a flash of white light and I heard a deep low sound, lower than the lowest key on a piano. I went down on one knee and lost consciousness briefly as the blinding white light went to black. When I came to, shortly after that, I was still on one knee and I thought someone had tried to put me in a playful headlock and missed. My male friends were always play-wrestling and roughhousing, and though I hadn't expected it of Angela's date, he was probably just trying to be friendly.

Just as I stood to ask Angela and her friend what had happened, there was a second punch to my head from another direction, then a third. I was knocked from side to side and I lost my footing each time, but now I could see Angela and her date in front of me and I knew it wasn't him. Were my friends really just standing there while this happened? "Goddamn it, help!" I shouted. They stood motionless and I noticed that Angela's mouth was shaped in a perfect O and she had this wild, horrified look in her eyes. Her date simply threw his hands in the air, turned, and walked away. I fell to the ground. While I lay prone on the sidewalk, the attackers rifled through the pockets of my leather jacket. I saw Angela run inside the restaurant — I hoped she was looking for someone to come help. I managed to grab one of the men by the crotch and squeeze with all my might, then I bit him on the thigh. If I was going to die, someone was going to have a scar to remember me by. A different guy then kicked me in the back of the head in retaliation and shouted an antigay epithet. Punches rained down on me from all directions. It felt like my head was on fire. I didn't know how many men were attacking me, as I couldn't get far enough away to gain perspective. I thought it might be a gang.

In the chaos of the mugging, they never once looked in my back jeans pocket, where I'd put my wallet with the two hundred dollars tucked inside. Frustrated, they settled for the jacket, ripping it off my body and then running down the street. I caught a glimpse of them and knew it was the same two men who'd been in the bar with us. I'd felt no fear while they followed us down the stairs — they towered over me, but they'd looked so clean-cut and strait-laced.

I struggled to my feet. Not only was I in a lot of pain, but I was having trouble getting my bearings. The world looked different: off kilter, dreamlike. Everything that moved had trails of colored light following close behind it. There were triangles and squares in repeating patterns wherever I looked, from the windows to the lampposts to the street signs. Angela came back outside, and though she'd been frozen in place during the attack, now she moved toward me in bizarre, stop-action frames. I rubbed my eyes. The glow of the streetlights seemed amplified. I could see the cars going by, little chipped shapes bouncing off their hoods.

I stumbled into the restaurant and managed to shout, "Call 911!" while I attempted to catch my breath.

"If you want to call 911 you'll have to go somewhere else," said one of the waitresses. Angela was by my side and as frustrated and shocked as I was. Neither of us had a cell phone.

Could this be real? I felt like it was a nightmare. I told the waitress that I'd just been attacked by two of their patrons and that they needed to preserve their plates and silverware and glasses for fingerprints. She told me to leave. I asked for the slips of paper from the karaoke registry that might have their names on it. She pointed to the garbage cans.

I clearly wasn't getting anywhere, and both my head and my back were killing me, but I had a little bit of good luck—it wasn't far to Tacoma General Hospital. The doctors took x-rays and did CT scans and found a baseball-size bruise on my kidney. I would have blood in my urine for the next few days, they said, but they released me that night. They figured I had a profound concussion. Little did they know how profound.

Angela had followed me to the hospital, and of course her date was long gone by then. She vowed never to see him again. I gave her a ride home even though the doctors had advised me not to drive. All the way there, I couldn't believe the light show of shapes and colors before my eyes. It was all I could do to stay in my lane.

When I got back to my house I couldn't sleep. I lay awake reliving the incident over and over, but in my mind I killed them every time.

In one scenario I had a box cutter from work in my pocket and slit their throats; in another, the cops showed up and shot them dead. It was totally unlike me to have violent thoughts but I'd never been so profoundly physically and mentally violated in my life.

I was angry with myself for not figuring out what was going on from the beginning. My intuition had told me something was off twice that night — when I noticed how seedy the location was and when I caught the bartender staring at my wallet — but I completely ignored the signs.

The next day I woke to more incredible visual phenomena. When I used the sink and took a shower that morning, I saw lines emanating out perpendicularly from the flow of the water. The lines extended beyond the basin and the tub and I quickly stepped back for a moment, since some of the lines were heading toward me. At first I was startled, and worried for myself, but it was so beautiful that I just stood in my slippers and stared. I also felt some vertigo as I tried to walk around in the midst of the light show. Despite how upsetting and disorienting it was, I forced myself to clean up, get dressed, and return to the bar to ask, yet again, for help in learning the identities of my attackers. They stonewalled me, just like they had the night before, and it made me feel victimized all over again.

But I trusted that I would recover. I had no idea that I'd left the old Jason behind, lying in a heap on that sidewalk.

CHAPTER FOUR

Gray Matter

N MY MIND, I'd play back the attack beginning with the last happy moments when I was whole, before the painful impact with its flash of light, the impossibly low piano note, and then the blackness. I watched myself crumple to the ground. In the days after the attack, I continued to relive the mugging over and over again. I obsessed over every detail, trying to remember exactly where I was struck and how many times. Soon I began to see it as though I were watching from outside myself.

I began researching traumatic brain injuries (often referred to as TBIs) online. Soon the brutal narrative of that night, still on a re-play loop in my obsessive mind, was overlaid with new information at every critical point. A new, richer story emerged as I began to come to grips with the reality of what had happened.

As I exited the bar, just before the mugging, my healthy three-pound brain was floating in a bath of cerebrospinal fluid, moving ever so slightly with each step I took. Inside my brain, some of my one hundred billion neurons were busy talking to one another thanks to an information network that's more complex than any computer's on earth. Electrochemical signals were flying through my brain, some at speeds of more than two hundred miles per hour, across a web of nerve fibers that if stretched out would measure about one hundred thousand miles. The nerve fibers responsible for sending out all these transmissions are called axons, and they look like long, thin tails on the ends of neurons. A protective coating called myelin encases the axons and helps keep the communications flowing at top speed.

Thanks to all this brain activity, I was able to instantaneously interpret and navigate the world around me as I left the bar — accurately calculating the height of the steps I walked down so I wouldn't trip, pulling my leather jacket tighter around me in response to the cool night air, and, of course, replaying my rocking Bon Jovi performance in my mind. Believe me, there was nothing extraordinary about what was going on inside my brain. It's just what average brains do on a daily basis.

The first punch hit the back of the right side of my head, but that initial impact, or what brain experts call the coup, was only the beginning of the problem. My brain was likely propelled by that force to the other side of my head — the contrecoup.

During the mugging, my brain likely had at least two points of impact for each blow, but that's not the only damage that occurred. Brains, I have since learned, are not hard and rubbery, as I once thought, but rather the consistency of tofu or Jell-O, and my fragile brain was slammed violently into a number of sharp, bony ridges protruding from the interior of my skull, causing it even more harm. In addition, there were injuries right down to the cellular level.

Scientists now know that when the brain ricochets inside the skull, it can stretch or even tear the myelin sheaths that protect axons. It's the same mechanism that causes whiplash in a car accident. In an accident, the head jerks forward and then back, overstretching or tearing the muscles and ligaments in the neck. I suffered a kind of brain whiplash, overstretching the delicate structures inside my head, an injury that can kill neurons or damage them so badly they are no longer able to communicate.

Despite the shock of what had happened and of my new perceptions, I was filled with intense curiosity and began researching on the Internet other cases of concussions and TBI. I immersed myself in the stories of what happened to other people in my situation. I wasn't sure why I now had such an aptitude for research. And for the first time, my interests didn't lie in thrills or the rush of my social life. Was this some temporary side effect of the beating I took? Unfortunately, I didn't have the money for the medical testing necessary to get more answers. This isolation also had another layer: I was now afraid to leave the house.

What I learned from my personal research painted a stunning picture of what happened to my brain the night I was attacked. I knew it was tragic, but it was also fascinating at every turn. In some ways, it was like passing a terrible accident on the road. I was afraid to look and at the same time unable to turn away.

I was seeing the most bizarre things. When I extended my hand and then withdrew it, it was like watching a slow-motion film. I saw an image on the television of light glistening on a lake, and it was as though the light points also emanated from the screen — they grew larger than the actual image. I was obsessed with every shape in my house, from the rectangles of the windows to the curvature of a spoon. The house itself seemed to fall away as a whole and become just a collection of shapes. The sudden importance of geometry — whether in the environment or in my visions — felt at once invasive and awe-inspiring.

I realized there must have been some misfiring going on because there were physical symptoms. It began a day or so after the mugging: I was lying in bed, and my right foot started to vibrate. It felt like someone had laid a violin or a small guitar on top of my foot and started strumming it. The vibrations went over the top of my foot like waves of different tones; I could feel the change in frequency in my skin and deep in my muscles. It was almost as though I could hear the notes the imaginary instrument was playing because the depths and vibrations varied as though they were music, like the way it feels at a very loud live music event, only much deeper in my musculature. It continued for longer than any song; it was more like an entire symphony. Several weeks later, I became so worried about this that I left the safety of my house and went to the doctor. I was sent for a magnetic resonance imaging (MRI) scan one Friday, and the neurologist who ordered the test told me my symptoms might be due to multiple sclerosis, Parkinson's disease, or Lou Gehrig's disease, among other disorders, and he'd have the results on Monday. I spent the weekend frantic that something would show up to confirm I had one of these devastating illnesses.

On Monday, a nurse from the doctor's office phoned and said the MRI showed no evidence of any of these diseases. She said it was likely that the twitches and tremors, which had also started to affect my arms and my legs and even my tongue, were a result of the concussion I'd suffered during the mugging. She couldn't say how long they might last, but she did say they could stop at any time and were not considered dangerous. The condition was called benign fasciculation syndrome, a fancy name for involuntary muscle tics. These twitches can happen in any skeletal muscle in the body and are sometimes visible through the skin. I sat one day watching the waves of them ebb and flow through the back of my hand. Though they are often found in otherwise healthy people, they can interfere with the quality of life. Magnesium deficiency is a common cause of involuntary muscle twitches, but my level was apparently normal.

I felt so strange with my visual impressions and physical tremors that all I wanted to do was retreat to my home. I felt compelled to sit alone just pondering things, stuck in the puzzlement of what I was becoming. It was a strange fate to have mobility of body but not of mind — my mind, while opening up whole new worlds to me, was like an anchor keeping me still and thinking for the first time in my life.

I continued to obsess over the accident and what might have happened if things had gone differently. What if Angela hadn't needed a ride that night? What if I'd said no to going out? Why did we choose that particular place at that particular time on that particular night? What if my Alaska crew of guy friends had been with me to bail me out? For the first time in my life, I tried to do the math on the statistical likelihood of a specific event occurring. I don't even know how I realized it had to do with math or probability, but I did. Other things in life suddenly had math behind them as well — I found myself counting my steps as I crossed the living room or went up the stairs to my house. I started thinking about the infinitesimally small chance that I had even been born, given all the millions of circumstances that had had to be aligned, from the Big Bang to the migrations and marriages of my thousands of ancestors. I now wanted to know how everything worked. I had deep questions about the mysteries of the universe and my place in it, and the feeling was a bit euphoric.

What was most peculiar to me about some of these thoughts was how fresh they felt. I sensed they weren't inspired by old memories of teachings I'd forgotten; they resonated from somewhere deeper than that.

As wondrous as my new abilities seemed to be, the drawbacks that accompanied them were plentiful. Many brain-injury victims change for the worse, not the better, and I was already showing signs of some of the negative effects. I had no idea at the time how common brain injuries were, but I soon discovered that I was just one of an estimated 1.7 million Americans annually who suffered TBIs. I was shocked to learn that about fifty thousand people died each year from brain injuries, and as many as ninety thousand developed some sort of lifelong disability. In fact, according to the

Centers for Disease Control (CDC), traumatic brain injury is the leading cause of death and permanent disability for Americans under forty-five.

I continued combing through the frightening statistics and found that survivors can experience a wide range of negative changes — mood swings, emotional imbalances, cognitive impairment, anger issues, poor concentration, and the deterioration of social skills. To their friends and families, they can come across as completely different people. The bad news didn't stop there. I also found that survivors are at increased risk of developing substance abuse, depression, phobias, psychotic disorders, and posttraumatic stress disorder (PTSD). The odds of any or all of these happening to me were enormous. I was already starting to notice some of the more common cognitive consequences of TBI: impaired judgment and difficulty with decision-making.

I noticed that I now didn't want to be around other people, but at the same time, I wished I had just one trusted person near me who could tell me exactly what to do — from what to eat for breakfast to how to handle the consequences of my injuries. I couldn't come to a decision about anything — even which shirt to wear when I got dressed in the morning. I worried about people not wanting to be around me if I began to exhibit an inability to relate. It's not always easy to tell if someone's had a brain injury; TBI survivors tend to look normal. But people with brain injuries can miss important social cues, like when a conversation is over or when someone is growing annoyed or uncomfortable.

I worried I was becoming another Phineas Gage, the railroad worker whose story I came across in my reading. On September 13, 1848, Gage was leading a group of men working for the Rutland and Burlington Railroad near Cavendish, Vermont. Gage was compacting blasting charges with a large iron rod when the powder exploded and propelled the rod through his head. It was an inch and a quarter thick and more than a yard in length. It pierced the side of his skull behind his left eye and then continued through, exiting out of the top of his head.

Gage miraculously recovered from the horrible wound and lived, but his personality transformed dramatically. In 1868, one of his doctors, John Martyn Harlow, wrote that the man who had previously been even-tempered, energetic, and well regarded by his peers was now "fitful, irreverent, indulging at times in the grossest profanity (which was not previously his custom)." Quite simply, wrote Harlow, he was "no longer Gage."

Reading about Phineas Gage made me worry. I walked over to the mirror and stared for a long time. I knew I'd become a different person, just like he had. And yet, parts of me were still the same. In the weeks after the mugging, I'd begun to lose weight and looked extremely tired, yes, but when I looked at my eyes, they were the same color and shape. How could they look the same when I was seeing so many new things?

Fortunately, I had something that Gage did not: access to advanced medical knowledge and high-tech brain-imaging tools. I'd had that one MRI scan for my fasciculations, which to my surprise had come back normal. I have since learned that it's not that unusual for an MRI to miss the type of damage associated with mild traumatic brain injury. MRIs do provide more detailed three-dimensional images of the brain than CT scans, which are typically used to detect skull fractures and life-threatening bleeding in the brain. But MRIs aren't sensitive enough to pick up damage at the microscopic or cellular level. Nowadays, there are more effective brain-imaging scans available, such as functional MRI (fMRI), which measures brain activity by showing detailed images of blood flow throughout the brain. This type of test probably could have detected changes in the way my brain functioned. Unfortunately, fMRI wasn't widely used at the time. I couldn't afford additional testing anyway, and I'd never heard of anything more advanced than a regular MRI, so I didn't pursue further studies.

Even the doctors responsible for my care at the time didn't recommend any other testing. In the medical community, there are agreed-upon protocols for severe brain injuries — say a bullet wound that leaves a gaping hole. But when it comes to treating closed-head, less traumatic injuries, like mine, there is a bit of a gray area. Despite the fact that my MRI was read as normal, my new impressions of the world persisted, and they were as astonishing as they were disturbing.

In the mugging, I had received three direct punches to the back and sides of my skull and at least one very hard kick to the back of it. My skull wasn't fractured, probably owing to bone being one of the strongest materials found in nature.

Bone is, ounce for ounce, stronger than steel. Even though the eight bones that make up the human skull average only about a quarter of an inch in thickness, some parts of the skull are estimated to be able to withstand a force of twelve hundred to fourteen hundred pounds. Research shows that Olympic and professional boxers are capable of delivering blows that top one thousand pounds of force per square inch. Lucky for me, the guys who assaulted me were likely delivering only about sixty to eighty-five pounds of force per square inch, which is the average for a human punch. The kicks to my head were probably about three and a half times stronger, but still within the ability of my skull to withstand them. But that doesn't mean that nothing devastating happened inside my head.

The mugging did physical damage to my brain, but it also did psychological damage, a result of being the victim of a violent crime. I was warned I might experience some posttraumatic stress disorder symptoms related to this, and as I read about it, I really began to recognize the feelings I was having. I was becoming afraid to leave my home and afraid to be around people. I couldn't explain it beyond the fact that people, even my friends, made me feel uncomfortable and suspicious.

From what I understand, it's completely normal to feel anxious, jumpy, or frightened for some time after something traumatic happens. But when those feelings don't go away or when they start interfering with everyday life, then it may be PTSD. To understand this better, I needed to look at what had been happening inside my body while I was being attacked.

As I walked out of the bar on the night of the mugging, my body was in a state of homeostasis, or internal equilibrium. But when I was attacked, a part of my brain called the hypothalamus sent out an SOS message, triggering my body's natural fight-or-flight stress response. A cascade of hormones, including adrenaline and cortisol, flooded into my bloodstream, causing my heart to beat faster and my breathing to quicken. My muscles tensed up so they were ready for action. And my liver started breaking down glycogen (a form of sugar) and converting it into glucose so I'd have the energy to either fight back or run for my life (that's why they call it the fight-or-flight response). I tried to fight back — remember, I bit that one guy on the thigh! Sometime after the mugging was over, this chemical surge subsided, and my body returned to its state of homeostasis.

The problem is that in some people, when a traumatic event occurs, the body's stress response system gets out of whack and gets stuck on high alert. Little things, like a door slamming or a telephone ringing, can trigger the fight-or-flight response. It's like you feel like you're still under attack even though you're in the comfort of your own living room. That's PTSD, and it comes with a laundry list of unpleasant symptoms, including flashbacks, insomnia, nightmares, being easily startled, and more. I found myself exhibiting some of the most classic PTSD symptoms: reliving the mugging over and over, avoiding situations that reminded me of the event, and feeling both numb and overstimulated at the same time.

It turns out that, according to the National Center for PTSD, there are about 7.7 million Americans who suffer from the condition. I was surprised to learn that not everyone who suffers a trauma gets PTSD. In fact, most people who live through some form of trauma don't develop the condition. Why are so many people able to handle the stress while others, like me, can't seem to get over it? Experts say that it depends in part on the intensity of the traumatic event as well as the amount of support a person gets afterward. But that's not all. Genetics and past traumas can also play a role in the likelihood of someone developing PTSD.

I was beginning to realize that my situation put me at higher risk for the condition. I had gotten injured in the mugging, felt like I had no control during the event, and wasn't getting adequate support in the aftermath. At the time, I was so laser-focused on the mugging as the trigger for my PTSD that I didn't even stop to think about how other life events might have contributed to the problem. It wasn't until much later that I would realize that my parents' numerous divorces and remarriages, the death of my infant son, and other family troubles might have had something to do with it too.

It helped to read about other people in the same situation, and I hoped that one day I would get the help I needed. Even though I knew that seeking help would be good for me, it wasn't enough to motivate me to act back then. I didn't want to leave the house — my fear was truly disabling.

Though I was very concerned for myself after reading about PTSD, I felt that the greater mystery was my new visions and abilities. I'd never heard of anyone who experienced the things that were happening to me. At the same time, I was also becoming fascinated by the greater cosmos and wondering how I, and my consciousness, fit into the whole universe. I even broke my self-imposed exile briefly and bought a telescope from Costco to look deeper into the galaxy; I peered out at the night sky from my darkened living room.

I was filled with questions about everything from outer space to my inner space. I wondered if there were even words to describe what was happening to me.

CHAPTER FIVE

Compounded Losses

I NITIALLY, SOME SERIOUS distractions kept me from having to face the profound changes my mind had undergone. My mother called the day after the mugging, and once I had relayed my own bad news, she told me my stepfather had lost his fight with cancer the same night that I was attacked. To lose my stepdad was a very deep blow. He may not have been my biological father, but he was the one stepfather of many I had who was as much a father to me as any man could be. He was a happy force and a stabilizing influence in my life from the age of twelve onward. My fractured family consisted of divorced biological parents with multiple remarriages between them, but this man, Captain Steve Smith, my hero, was not just passing through. He was a real father figure and mentor. I felt devastated and very much alone.

Captain Smith was a Special Forces operative in Vietnam who was shot down twice during his tour of duty. He liked to say stoically that he got a vasectomy courtesy of the Viet Cong during one of these attacks: a chopper he was in was shot at, and shrapnel from the artillery that blew off his pilot's head landed between his own legs. He managed to fly the chopper ninety miles and get it to a safe area before it went down. The other time he was shot down in a helicopter, he found himself in a field surrounded by the enemy. Thrown from the vehicle, he nonetheless made it back through heavy fire to blow the chopper up, as it was carrying sensitive equipment. A friend of senators and high-ranking military officials, he instilled in me a strong work ethic.

He also gave me my first exposure to obsessive-compulsive disorder (OCD). Captain Smith ran such an orderly household that when dining-room chairs were moved to new positions, he made my brother and me rub out the previous marks in the carpeting. Even with this tic, he inspired me to be more self-sufficient. He did not give me a lot of material things, but he provided a strong example of personal responsibility and mettle. There would not be a funeral, my mother said — Captain Smith wanted to be remembered the way he had been.

He was the one person I probably needed most in the world right then, someone strong who would help me find the men who had done this to me. If anyone could have found my attackers and brought them to justice, it was Steve. I let that thought guide me in my next move.

That day, the day after the mugging, I called a few friends and we gathered to make posters stating that the karaoke bar was involved in the cover-up of a violent crime. We drove to the bar and marched out front until a television news crew showed up. Between the journalists covering the story and my group informing several dozen patrons showing up at the business what had happened the night before — several of them turned on their heels and left; some went in and gave the management an earful — we eventually got the owner to come outside. At first he was angry and called the police on us, thinking that we were disturbing the peace and that we were not allowed to protest. The police came and said that we were not breaking any laws, shook my hand, and left. Minutes afterward, the restaurant owner provided me with the names and addresses of the attackers and asked us to leave. We did.

For the next five days I tried to get police to respond to my calls about the incident, with no success. Just two weeks after my mugging, Tacoma police chief David Brame would shoot and kill his wife and then himself in front of their kids while seated in the family car in a grocery-store parking lot. Eleven months later, the FBI would descend on the city to investigate allegations of police corruption and illegal business transactions by government officials. To say that the crime against me happened in a strange policing environment is an understatement. I didn't know what was going on at the time; I just knew I was getting nowhere asking for help. So I did surveillance on the attackers' home myself and found they were roommates and that they were packing up to move. I was so angry, I pulled my car up on their lawn just four feet from their front door to announce my arrival. I knocked on their door and told all who passed what the occupants had done to me. I told neighbors to call the police; the men were wanted for a violent crime. One of the assailants answered the door and began to shake and stutter as he tried to stare me down. A squad car showed up, and the police questioned him with me by their side. This time, the police treated the situation differently. The man admitted to the crime, claiming they were drunk that night. It came to light that two women employees of the bar, one of whom was the bartender who'd eyed my wallet, were dating the thugs. He was arrested on the spot and the other one was tracked down later that day.

I collapsed with relief when I heard the police had both men in custody, but my relief was short-lived. With the capture of my attackers accomplished, I now had time to think about what had happened to me and to my stepfather, and a depression began to set in. I was so immobilized by grief I took some time off from Planet Futon to regroup. At first I thought it would be just a couple of weeks.

Then weeks turned into months. Three months into my isolation, I got a phone call from my brother John's live-in girlfriend, Keri. It was the day after Christmas, and I'd barely acknowledged the holiday. "We had an argument," she explained when she called; she was checking to see if I had heard from John. "He put out the garbage and tracked in a bunch of water. I yelled at him and he said, 'I can't do anything right!' before grabbing some pills and a blanket and walking out the door. I'm really worried. I think something terrible has happened." He'd been missing almost twenty-four hours.

"You know my brother," I countered. "He's walked out before and he's always made his way to a nice hotel. John likes his creature comforts. He'll come back eventually."

I was pretty sure John would turn up, but I still spent some time over the next couple of weeks working down a list of phone numbers of my brother's friends and associates. He'd never been gone more than a week before. Sometimes when I looked at the phone numbers, I'd see different shapes for each number. I'd see cubes for individual numbers, and if I stared at the whole strand of numbers, these big crystal grids would form before me or in my mind's eye. I would lose myself pondering this bizarre imagery for a while, then snap myself out of it and go back to working down the list. I was as determined to find my brother as I had been to find the men who mugged me. Several times I called people at inappropriate hours, unaware of what day of the week it was, much less what time. I had not yet returned to work, I had no real routine, and I was beginning to lose track of time. No one seemed to have any information.

My mind was also flooded by memories of my brother. Two things occurred to me: First, my long-term memory was apparently intact. I could remember back to our days as toddlers very clearly. And second, these memories were smooth as they played, like movies in my mind. My present-day perceptions were choppy and stop-action and overlaid with strange shapes, but the memories appeared just as I used to see the world. I would get lost in them over and over. It was much less exhausting than considering the present. They also brought me back to a time when John and I were close. I remembered the day I almost drowned and John tried to save me. I wanted to repay the brother who had rushed to my aid when we were small, even though we'd drifted apart in recent years. I picked up the list of phone numbers and worked down it again. No one had heard a thing.

One morning I woke with the belief that John was dead. It hit me like a truck. My mind was different since the attack, and I didn't always react in a timely fashion. I couldn't even choose among various cans of corn on a supermarket shelf back then, and I still tend to ask people around me for help with decisions. Before the mugging, I always knew what I wanted and I'd walk through walls to get it; now, except for the emergencies of solving my mugging and finding my brother, I just wanted to hide behind walls. Keri had immediately known that something was very wrong when John left, and I had shrugged it off.

One day, I lay in bed thinking about my brother being dead, my stepfather being dead, and what had happened to me. Suddenly I snapped.

I jumped up and pulled my blankets off the bed and frantically ran for my toolbox. I took out the hammer and went window to window nailing the blankets over the frames to block out the world. When I used up those blankets, I went to the linen closet and got more blankets and sheets and worked my way around the rest of the house. My heart was pounding in my chest and I began to sweat. I was so manic that I tripped over the fabric a few times in my haste.

The last clouds I saw, before covering up the final window, had discrete components, a stream of still pictures, each one slightly different than the last, as the cumulus forms changed shape in the wind. I paused momentarily to consider them, teetering on my stepstool with vertigo from the impression, and then I hurriedly got back to my mission. In my altered perception, motion still occurred in stop-action frames. It was as though the great animator of us all had pulled the veil back to show me the individual sketches that, when streamed, gave movement to everything.

I wondered where John's body was, and if I hadn't been so afraid of stepping outside my house, I'd have conducted a search myself. Terrible images of his lifeless form began flashing through my mind. I was reeling from the compounded losses and overwhelmed by a need to hide. After I finished with the blankets and sheets, I checked the chains on the doors multiple times and wedged brooms and bats against the undersides of the doorknobs as early-warning devices. I looked inside all the rooms, even opening the closets and pushing things aside to make sure no one was lurking in them. Then I repeated the sweep, somewhere between five and ten times in all.

I was aware of my blossoming OCD during this frenzy. In addition to checking and rechecking the locks, I'd been checking over and over to make sure the stove was off, washing my hands raw, and peering out the windows suspiciously several times a day. Unlike the other things going on with me, OCD was something I'd heard of; I knew it was related to anxiety, but I was powerless to stop it. I became a hyperaware sentry in my own home.

In the days that followed, in my darkened cave, I decided I would stop going to work at Planet Futon altogether and live off my savings. While my dad was concerned about me, he was also very upset that I was quitting, and he tried to talk me into going back. I couldn't snap out of my agoraphobia. One of our salespeople took over the management of the store. When I needed groceries, I slipped out at three in the morning and filled the car to overflowing so I wouldn't have to go out again for several weeks, checking my rearview mirror constantly on the way home to see if I was being followed. The light of the grocery store, bright by anyone's standards, was blinding to me. I seemed to be developing photosensitivity from my isolation in the house. All people seemed suspicious to me after the attack, and the people in the store just jabbered on and on nonsensically. Their mundane world of appointments and coupon-clipping and idle talk on the checkout line didn't interest me. In retrospect, I realize I must have seemed pretty strange to them — looking over my shoulder constantly and scooting from the aisle if anyone else came down it. I mostly subsisted on Pop-Tarts and breakfast cereals and frozen pizza rolls. I'd never really been one to cook because I spent most of my nights out in clubs that served bar food or dinner. I hated going to the supermarket, and if I could have forgone food altogether and stayed in my isolation, I would have. But I was afraid to have food delivered by strangers, and home delivery was too expensive for my budget anyway, so the shopping trips were a concession, an unavoidable risk. Though I formerly had had a healthy appetite, now it was gone; I ate very little, rationing my provisions to postpone those forays into the now-surreal market. I didn't care what anything tasted like. I would eat once a day, just to prevent hunger pangs. My once-muscular frame began to wither away.

Before I retreated permanently to my house I'd gone to the barbershop and said, "Cut it all off!" My eyes started hurting from the hours I spent researching online, so I dug out an old pair of reading glasses and began wearing them all the time. I looked in the mirror one day and didn't recognize myself. I wanted to hide from that realization as much I wanted to hide from the outside world.

Perhaps my darkened enclave was a womb of sorts; a cocoon where I could transform before I went out into the world as a new person. I didn't know how to be that new person yet. Was this person a crime victim? Was he a brain-injury sufferer? Would the new visions I was having define who I became? I was able to compare the me from before the mugging and the me after it, and they didn't match up, which was very confusing to me. I had trouble identifying with the fun-loving young man I knew I'd been before the attack. Now I felt like I had developed a completely different personality, changes well beyond the new visual abilities. I thought back to Phineas Gage, the brain-injury survivor who was described as being "no longer Gage." Was I no longer Jason?

It was hard to let go of the old me. In the beginning, I mourned the loss of my old familiar feeling of self, which was only a memory now. I'd been a popular guy with lots of friends and I'd had plenty of fun times, from going out on dates to clubbing. I couldn't imagine doing any of that now, though sometimes I still wanted to be out there engaging with the world. I remember seeing a weather report on television during that time showing people playing at a swimming pool. Part of me wanted to be out there having fun, but the rest of me just couldn't move to do it. I thought enviously about cases of amnesia I'd heard about. It would be so much easier to accept this new me if I didn't have to remember who I once was.

I took out some old Polaroids and marveled at this other self from the past; gone were the muscle T-shirts that best displayed my bulging biceps, and gone was the spiky fade haircut. The man holding these images had adopted a studious, bespectacled, but toned-down look, and I wasn't quite sure why. I wasn't the carefree boy in those photos any longer. I had too many unanswered questions about my brain and consciousness and reality.

While I couldn't change who I now was, there were steps I could take to better enable me to face the world as my new self. I decided to learn as much as I could about my medical situation and hopefully take small steps toward embracing the diagnosis, whatever it might be. At the same time, I knew I needed to learn all I could about science and math to help me understand the strange new phenomena before my eyes.

I was seeing shapes and grids that I couldn't understand, as well as bright horizontal lines that would appear from moving objects. At first, I wondered if they were hallucinations. I'd never seen anything so strange and beautiful. But in my core, I felt the visions might be more profound than that. Perhaps they were manifestations of deeper patterns that had always been present in nature but that had been hidden from me up till now. They certainly opened up the world in a new way. It was as though I'd lived all my life in a Magic Eye poster, seeing only the obvious picture; now the hidden image was *all* I could see. I began to see and think about the geometry of everything. The mysteries of the universe were beckoning a man who had never even thought about them before.

I was unaware of this at the time, but in the silent recesses of my skull, my brain was working to heal itself, forming new neuronal connections to compensate for the ones that had been damaged. As my interests began to change and my personality moved from outgoing to bordering on antisocial, my brain was actually recovering in a miraculous way. This updated wetware, as some scholars and theorists refer to the human brain, would go on to make me capable of the biggest intellectual leaps I had ever taken. It would go on to be my bright side. But first, it locked me away from the rest of the living world.

If there was a consolation to my growing isolation, it was that my inner life was now filled with wonder. My vision was overlaid with rays of light, floating interlocking squares, and multiple frames of images of things in motion. It was as if the blows to my head had opened a window onto a geometric realm that had previously been painted shut. Many of the images I saw would turn out to correspond to concepts from physics that I had never studied. Theories of my own about the way things worked, particularly regarding movement and time, began percolating.

Clearly, something about me had drastically changed as a result of the attack. The gregarious old me, in search of the next good time, now found himself steeped in profound and serious thought all day. I'd be deep in contemplation, and the rare visitor I let in would walk up to me and I wouldn't even see him. The blows had changed me fundamentally. It seemed impossible, but I actually felt smarter, yet more and more isolated.

I could not stop thinking about geometry. I retreated into a pristine world of mathematics and cosmology — it was easy to ponder the heavens from inside my darkened house. My brain wouldn't turn off. *Everything* became related to geometry. I barely noticed my obsessive counting anymore. My brain felt full, bursting with thoughts and images. It wasn't just a form of escape, though there was that. I was unable to stop paying attention to the smallest details of the world that I had previously never noticed. I was overwhelmed by the wonder of it all.

Sometimes I pondered the new workings of my brain and tried to figure out where John was simultaneously. My addled gray matter had grown expansive, capable of multitasking — even when the mysteries were as enormous as these. It felt like my brain couldn't fit inside my skull anymore. It was as though the blows I'd received on that sidewalk opened my head and freed its contents. It was now oceanic in proportion. Life had a before-and-after quality. There were the forms and impressions before the mugging and after it. Before it, everything had seemed so large relative to my own size and self; afterward, I sometimes felt like a giant looking through a microscope.

The phone was my only lifeline to my fractured family; my mother was still living in Alaska, and my father had moved to Illinois. With my only sibling, John, gone, it was very easy for me to hide how dire things were. My family and friends didn't realize what was going on for a while because my phone manner was usually upbeat. My mother never got mad when I telephoned at all hours, and she would ask me to describe what I saw. My dad, however, got one too many late-night calls and took to saying, "Jesus Christ, Jason, do you know what time it is?" before I started talking.

My friend Angela, present the night of the mugging, tried desperately to get me out of my isolation. She phoned repeatedly and asked me to come out with her and our friends. I always declined. So one day she showed up at the house. I reluctantly let her inside.

"You need to take down those blankets, go take a shower, and come out with me," she announced. "Enough already — it's been weeks. You can't live like this."

"I don't want to go anywhere. I just want to be left alone," I told her.

"You need to be with people. This isn't normal, Jason." She was beginning to get angry.

"You're not in this situation — how could you understand?"

"If you stay in your house, that's them winning!" she yelled. "There will be a lot of people there tonight. You'll feel safe!"

I exploded. I can't remember raising my voice so fiercely to any-one — it just wasn't my nature, either before or after the mugging. But I'd heard enough. "Well, there were a lot of people around the night I was attacked, including you, and none of you did a damn thing — you just stood there. I'm not going. Now, get out!" I showed her the door. After that, I wouldn't even answer the doorbell. My loved ones tried to coax me from my cave from afar, but I seldom let anyone visit me. The one exception was my young daughter, Megan. But that didn't mean our visits were normal.

The doorbell would ring, and even if I was expecting my five-year-old, I'd have to make sure it was actually her. I'd tiptoe cautiously toward the front door and then peek out the side of the blanket covering the window closest to it, straining to look down at an angle toward what would be the height of my little brunette daughter. If her saucer-large blue eyes met mine and I was sure it was her and no one else, I'd remove the bat I'd propped against the door and quickly unbolt the locks, then open the door just wide enough for her to squeeze through. The less time the door was open and the smaller the angle, the greater my sense of security. I wouldn't even pause to wave at Michelle, who always dropped her off. Megan knew the drill and would rush in. She'd drop her book bag, fling her arms wide open, and run toward me for a hug, but I'd recoil. I always did when she was coming straight from kindergarten. Megan hadn't figured out why, she just knew her dad was different now. It wasn't her; it was that I knew she'd been in contact with strangers and their germs all day.

I'd tell her to go wash up and she'd dutifully run off. I often wondered if it seemed like a game to her, because she giggled as she skipped. Once I could hear the water running in the bathroom, I'd find my bottle of antibacterial lotion and pump it around ten times into my hand. I'd taken to buying this instead of washing my hands until they bled. I'd slather it on my arms, my hands, my neck, and my face — every bit of skin was covered that might be exposed to any lingering germs from the kindergarten class.

Megan would reenter the room, shaking her hands dry as she approached. "Are you shiny enough now, Daddy?" she'd ask, and I'd nod.

Then I could finally hug my daughter.

CHAPTER SIX

New Gifts

AS A CHILD, I had a vast seashell collection. My prized piece was a brown polka-dot nautilus that had been varnished. How many hours had I stared at this store-bought addition to the other shells, most of which I'd found on vacation beaches with my family? I had liked it because it was so clean and glossy. In childhood imaginings, staring at that shell, I saw myself going round and round the spirals like a slide, the spiral never ending and the sound of the ocean echoing in the white halls of my seashell amusement ride. I wondered about my favorite shell's previous life under the sea and the creature that had inhabited it. How deep underwater had it lived? What had it eaten? Where had it been in its travels? How had it died? How could it be so utterly perfect living in the murky depths until some fisherman or a crashing wave tossing it ashore had led it to me?

One day, I was bingeing on information again, glued to my chair, sitting in front of the computer in my house for the fourth straight hour. I'd been searching for the repetitive geometric forms I was

seeing before my eyes when a nautilus shell appeared in the re-
trieved entries on my screen. I clicked on it immediately. There
was something at once familiar about the spiraling natural form.
I'd seen it in my childhood prized possession, but I'd also seen it in
my morning coffee as I stirred; I'd watched it every day as the water in the sink went down the drain. And one of the new images I
saw repeatedly was a spiral out in space. I often wondered about
its seemingly infinite reach and how smaller parts of it echoed the
larger parts. But I hadn't connected that outer-space shape to the
nautilus, much less to other things I was noticing in nature, until
now. As I read on, I learned that these shapes were known as fractals, a word I'd never heard before. Fractals are the fundamental,
repetitive geometric building blocks of everything in the known
universe, from seashells to the leaves and trees and mountains and
even to lightning. The pull of this newfound discovery was strong.
It seemed to signal to me that my visions could be something more
than the hallucinations of a brain-injury survivor. It felt like the beginning of a way back to sanity.

It all seemed to relate to something I'd seen during one early-
morning grocery-store run. There was a leafy tree with a branch
overhanging the roadway. The leaves became virtually see-through
in the glow from my headlights. Each leaf seemed to have its own
trunk and branches running through it, mirroring the tree as a
whole. I stared in wonder, and then I held my own hand up. I was
captivated and quickly flicked on the car's overhead light to be sure.
The veins of my hands branched out under my pale skin like those
of the leaves. The tiny wrinkles on my hand also seemed to be a repetitive pattern. My fingers seemed an echo of my arm, my arm an
echo of the trunk of my own body. *Why have I never noticed this
before?* I thought. I now had respect for the smallest things and was
filled with a sense of wonder about the world at large, despite my
ongoing fear of it. And as quickly as it had come on, my epiphany
passed, overtaken by the paranoia that someone would recognize

me with the car light on and try to harm me. I flicked the light off and continued driving.

I learned all I could about the fractal nature of the seashell and began researching the budding branch of mathematics known as fractal geometry. It was a very young discipline, developed in the 1970s by IBM researcher Benoit Mandelbrot and popularized in the 1980s after the publication of his book *The Fractal Geometry of Nature.* Why is fractal geometry so much more amazing than the stuff most of us learned in school? Textbook Euclidean geometry is what's used to measure or create smooth shapes — think of the clean edges of a high-rise building, the sleek lines of a countertop, or the symmetrical arch of a bridge. But it tends to fall short when one attempts to measure or reproduce the rough shapes found in nature, such as clouds, craters, or those coastlines I mentioned earlier. Mandelbrot's fractal geometry finally gave us a way to explore and understand the natural roughness in the world around us.

Mandelbrot came up with the concept of fractals while at IBM, where, amid all the number crunching and analysis, he began noticing repeating patterns within the data. He applied a simple mathematical formula, which has since become known as the Mandelbrot set, to the patterns he detected. I know that not everybody is as enthralled with fractal geometry and math as I am, but I can't help but share the actual formula. I think even math-averse people would have to admit that it looks surprisingly simple: $z_{n+1} = z_n^2 + C$. Where it gets tricky is that it involves complex numbers (a complex number is made up of two real numbers and one imaginary number). And to complicate things even more, every time you solve for z, you plug that new value back into the equation recursively and build it out, so the results never end. It can go on literally to infinity.

Things really got exciting when Mandelbrot put the powerful computing technology at IBM to work, letting the computers apply the formula over and over and over again — more times than any human possibly could. Next, he used the new technology to plot out a visual representation of the formula. The result? A breathtaking image of a fractal so intricately detailed that I could look at it on my computer and hit the zoom button ten times — or, if my computer would let me, a thousand, a million, or even a billion times — and see smaller and smaller subsets of similar but not quite identical patterns. Because of the Mandelbrot set's intricate patterns and never-ending nature, experts have said that the set may be the most complex of all mathematical objects.

The Mandelbrot set has captured popular imagination, outside of the realm of mathematics, for many reasons. For one thing, when plotted out, it's a very beautiful image. In a 2010 TED talk, Mandelbrot explained that depending on the specific numbers he plugged into the formula, the computers spit out shapes of "such complication, such harmony, and such beauty." He was absolutely right. I stared at the paisley- and ice-crystal-like images I found online and was awestruck and inspired. For some people, the Mandelbrot set is a glimpse into the infinite nature of the universe. Others see it as a way to find order in our chaotic world. Still others consider it a representation of the similarity shared by everything and everyone on this planet.

For me, it was a reflection of what was going on in my own mind — on a smaller scale, of course. Perhaps my mind wasn't processing what it saw on the same infinite scale Mandelbrot found, but I do think that what I experience is somehow a reflection of his work. Just as the Mandelbrot set reflects the universal order of things in nature (it has been referred to as "God's thumbprint"), I believe what I'm seeing is the very essence of ourselves and our universe.

One day I watched a documentary called *The Colours of Infinity.* It featured Mandelbrot and was hosted by the great science and science fiction writer Sir Arthur C. Clarke, who may be best known for cowriting the screenplay for the film *2001: A Space Odyssey*. Of course, I loved learning more about fractals, but what was most astounding to me was an interview with Michael Fielding Barnsley of Great Britain. A mathematician and author, he founded a company called Iterated Systems Incorporated and works on fractal models that can be applied to technology and even medicine. It occurred to me for the first time that while my visions were nice to look at, they might also have useful applications.

The deeper I looked into the application of fractals, the more I felt that what I was seeing wasn't so alien after all. Mandelbrot himself said in the documentary that humans might have discovered his set at any point in human history, given its organic nature and the simplicity of the math behind it. However, it wasn't until the powerful computers of the late twentieth century were able to plot millions of results that anyone could see it in all its complexity. Still, fractals can be seen in everything from ancient carpets from the Far East to Islamic tile work to Western stained-glass windows. In Mandelbrot's TED talk, he mentioned that even the Eiffel Tower in Paris had a fractal aspect to it. He suggested that its creator, Gustave Eiffel, was "intuitively" familiar with fractals. Had artists and architects through the ages seen the things I was now seeing? I knew that before my injury, I had noticed repeating patterns in the ragged edges of coastlines and in ice crystals, but now I was seeing repetitive geometric images in my own mind. Learning about fractals and the Mandelbrot set validated my belief that my new visions were giving me a firsthand look at the secrets of the universe. And yet this breakthrough, this glimmer of hope, still happened in darkness, behind the blankets I'd tacked up to my windows.

One month turned into one year, a year into two, two years into three, my darkened hovel lit only by the persistent, incandescent visions in my mind, the TV, and the computer monitor. Had someone peered in, he or she would have seen a man very much alone in his thoughts and research, a hermit who had almost no connection to the outside world. After three years, I'd given up hope my brother would ever return. I was missing now too, in my own way, having turned deep inside myself. It was hard to tell if I'd emerge from this self-imposed exile, but I was too obsessed with these new patterns in the universe to really care. This was my life now — I was drawn deep into the infinite and fractal spiral of my own mind.

Interruptions from the outside world were few and far between. My visits from Megan were always a high point, but my main companions in my seclusion were my memories, the TV, and the computer. They offered a safe connection to the outside world. My viewing and surfing habits were quite different than they'd been before, however. While I'd always had an interest in science fiction, I had never turned my attention to pure science. I used to watch football every Sunday and make a real occasion of it, popping corn and camping out on the sofa for hours with family and friends. Now I didn't care at all about my favorite teams. I found myself obsessed with any programming having to do with scientific research. Science fiction remained an interest too, but I was now more curious about the reality of science than the fantasy, with one exception.

I would set the alarm for three o'clock each morning, though sometimes I was already — or still — up, to watch my favorite TV show, *Farscape*. An Australian program that lasted four seasons, it featured the adventures of a character called John Crichton, an astronaut. He was part of a group trying to escape from corrupt authorities, called Peacekeepers. Crichton had accidentally flown through a wormhole and wanted to make his way back to Earth. At one point, to help Crichton get home, aliens implanted in his brain the ability to do higher math and physics. I was hooked. I had no delusions that my new abilities came from aliens, but like my hero, I was suddenly overwhelmed by what I knew and understood.

I too felt like a stranger in a strange land trying to find his way back home. That character, with whom I felt I had so much in common, was my only friend during a very lonely time. I was devastated when the series was canceled.

Then one night, about three years into my isolation, in the blue glow of the television, I stumbled on a program about a man named Daniel Tammet—a synesthete and autistic savant from England who was able to recite pi from memory to 22,514 places. This was even better than my scuttled hero John Crichton because Tammet was a real human being and he was interested in the same things I was. With his studious appearance and fair coloring, he even resembled the new me. At one point Tammet said he could do math so well because he could see it in shapes before his eyes.

I leaped from my chair and began jumping around the room. "That's it! That's what's going on with me. Oh my God! Someone else can see what I see!"

I rushed to my computer and Googled *Daniel Tammet, savant syndrome,* and a word I'd never heard before: *synesthesia.* I quickly learned that synesthesia is a sort of blending of the senses that can take many forms. Some people with synesthesia see colors when they look at numbers or letters—for example, *A* might be orange, *B* might be violet, and *C* might be lime green. Others see colors when they hear music. Still others may taste words or smell colors. In Tammet's case, he saw numbers as colors and shapes and said this helped him to remember them and calculate with great ease.

When I looked up savant syndrome, I found that, by definition, a savant is someone with a lot of knowledge about a particular subject or field. But the term often gets used to describe a person whose unusual aptitude for a specific subject or skill comes along with decreased abilities in other areas. Most savants, like the extremely high-functioning Tammet, are born that way. Not me. I was quickly realizing that my situation was far more rare. Experts called it sudden-onset savant syndrome or acquired savant syndrome. I read all

I could for many hours into the morning. Then I slept deeply, for the first time in months, with my face on the keyboard. The worry and confusion of the past three years had finally lifted a little.

Knowing I had a brain injury was pretty frightening. But sensing that I might have acquired synesthesia and savantism as a result was oddly exciting. Except I had no idea what those things were. After three years out of work, I definitely couldn't afford the required testing and medical advice, nor did I want to emerge from my house, so I set out to learn all I could on my own. I continued to mine that mother lode of all knowledge, the Internet.

I learned that at that time, there were only thirty documented cases of acquired savant syndrome on the entire planet, and none of the savants also had synesthesia. Could I be the only one in the world? I'd felt such pangs of recognition in seeing Tammet describe his own naturally occurring synesthesia and savantism, I was sure I must be right in thinking I had these syndromes. But I was not sure I wanted to be this new self, regardless of its rarity and its attractions.

Fortunately, I found I was living in a time of unprecedented research into both conditions. I had plenty of reading to do, as one Internet search led to another and then another. I discovered some very good journals and magazines reporting on both savantism and synesthesia, and I even found some YouTube interviews with savants and synesthetes. I watched video after video of people with one or the other of my two not-yet-diagnosed traits. I viewed them over and over, staring into the subjects' eyes, wondering what it was like to be them. To be me.

A few decades ago, if someone reported seeing synesthetic shapes for numbers and equations, doctors probably would have thought that person was hallucinating. But my injury and subsequent acquired synesthesia happened in the beginning of the twenty-first century and coincided with a surge of interest in this neurological topic. This newfound fascination was fueled by state-of-the-art brain-imaging technology, which, for the first time in history, allowed researchers to see various areas of the brain light up as it worked. When a person with synesthesia was shown numbers or letters while his brain was being scanned, scientists reported that two parts of the brain lit up; in a neurotypical subject, there was usually just a single area of response. That synesthesia was real and provable inspired many people to come out and be open about their odd abilities, even using them creatively. I discovered that many synesthetes were no longer afraid to explain and describe their experiences and were now employing various artistic media to express the sensations. As I sat at my computer desk in a corner of my living room, Google Images returned caches of their work. I stared at the paintings, sculptures, and collages, feeling waves of recognition at each form and color. I listened to music composed by synesthetes and read their poetry and prose. I took comfort in the fact that there were others out there expressing what they sensed synesthetically, though I'd yet to pick up a pencil and try it myself.

I learned that there are two types of synesthesia. The more common type, in which people see colors when they look at numbers or letters, is called perceptual, or lower, synesthesia. The type I suspected that I might have is less common and is known as conceptual, or higher, synesthesia. When I read or write a number, instead of seeing that number alone, in my mind's eye, I see a shape superimposed over it. Experts say that this type of conceptual synesthesia may involve areas within the parietal lobe, which is located near the top of the brain and is associated with a number of abilities related to language and math as well as with spatial cognition; that is, knowing where one is in space. People with injuries to the parietal lobe often have difficulty with math. My experience was quite the opposite — I felt these areas in my parietal lobe must be key to what was happening to me in a major way, as I was both synesthetic and adept at math, a subject about which I had previously known nothing. I learned that this area of the brain is also believed to be central to retrieving memories, which I found fascinating. I have always had a very good memory, and though my isolation skewed my sense of time, making it hard for me to keep track of dates and sequences of events, my recall for new facts and concepts had become better and more sharply focused since my injury.

I was pleased to learn that synesthesia is not always the result of an injury. Most people who have it are born with it, and many of them go on to become highly accomplished. The Nobel Prize–winning physicist and professor Richard Feynman was a synesthete; he saw colored letters. In his book *What Do You Care What Other People Think?*, he wrote: "When I see equations, I see the letters in colors — I don't know why. As I'm talking, I see vague pictures of Bessel functions from Jahnke and Emde's book, with light-tan *j*'s, slightly violet-bluish *n*'s, and dark brown *x*'s flying around. And I wonder what the hell it must look like to the students."

As I pored over all the descriptions of synesthesia I could find, I discovered that most of the definitions I came across referred to it as a condition, as if it were some sort of a medical ailment, mental-health problem, or disability. In fact, most synnies, as they call themselves, reject the word *condition*, or any other word with a negative connotation, to describe synesthesia. It certainly didn't feel like a disability to me. It was not only very beautiful but also helpful for my memory. I found I could remember numbers more easily due to the additional visuals.

I might not have had a blue Monday like Daniel Tammet or a dark brown *X* like Richard Feynman, but my brain was still doing backflips to come up with these shapes I saw when I thought of or looked at numbers.

The most interesting form of the phenomenon I read about was mirror-touch synesthesia. A person with mirror-touch synesthesia actually feels a physical sensation when he or she sees someone else being touched. The mechanism is related to the actions of mirror neurons, which we all have — they're the ones that make you flinch when you see someone get hit. Mirror-touch synesthesia might just be an exaggeration of that. Still, I was grateful I didn't have quite that much neurological activity. I thought it would be tiring to physically feel so much. But there was some research that showed that those mirror neurons activate the empathy response, and I recognized an increase in this in myself.

In my case, I felt more in touch with other people's emotions after my injury than I ever had before. Just being around other people, on the rare occasions I was, was overwhelming for me because I felt everything I felt *plus* what they felt too. If I spoke with someone who was having a bad day, I felt the anxiety of the person in my own stomach. The benefit of this was that I began to read people extremely well and I was much more compassionate than I had been. I noticed that people's body language really did reflect their inner thoughts and predict their behavior. I not only sensed what they were thinking but also began to feel their feelings. If they were happy, so was I. Their discomfort became my own. Occasionally, after spending time with others, I had to retreat and go somewhere quiet and dark so I could rest from human encounters for a while.

I learned that the new era of synesthesia research had begun despite the doubts of many medical researchers. Lawrence Marks, a professor of epidemiology and psychology at the Yale School of Public Health, pioneered some of the earliest modern research in synesthesia in the 1970s. In the 1980s, Richard Cytowic, a professor of neurology at George Washington University, in Washington, DC, looked into it using emerging brain-imaging technology. Both of them mentioned in interviews that they had to persevere despite the misgivings of their peers, who initially found the topic too far out. The doctors ultimately found enough hard evidence in case studies to continue, and they are now considered the fathers of modern synesthesia research. They launched a new era of scientific inquiry into the phenomenon, and it continues in dozens of learning institutions and labs around the world.

Before neuroimaging was widely available, Dr. Cytowic created several criteria to test people who claimed to have synesthesia. I read through the criteria and checked them against my own experiences. First, the ability must be automatic and involuntary. Check. Second, the images must be spatially extended, meaning perceived outside the body. That was certainly the case with mine. Third, the experiences must be consistent and simple. Well, mine were at least consistent. Fourth, the sensations needed to be vivid and memorable, even when recalled months later. That was also true for me, as I saw the same visions over years, not just months. And fifth, the perceptions needed to be experienced as real and undeniably true, causing an emotional response in the person experiencing them. If euphoria was an emotion, I could cross that element off the list with ease, I thought.

I felt all of these points matched my own reality, yet I could not find any examples of synesthetes who saw the things I did.

I kept searching for ways to verify and validate my self-diagnosis of synesthesia and eventually came across something called the Test of Genuineness (TOG). Developed in 1987 by a team of researchers including Simon Baron-Cohen, a professor of developmental psychopathology at Cambridge University in England, the TOG was designed to gauge how consistent a synesthete's response to a specific stimulus was. For example, does someone who sees an *A* as red *always* see it as red? Or is it sometimes purple or navy blue? Does a person who sees emerald green when she hears an F-sharp *always* see emerald green with that note? Or does it change? To find out, people took the TOG and then retook it several months later. The researchers found that people who had synesthesia typically scored from 70 to 90 percent in consistency. Among the nonsynesthetes, consistency was usually between 20 to 38 percent. I knew the images I saw in response to numbers or equations were consistent over time but I didn't seek out official testing.

Another really interesting test I learned about came from V. S. Ramachandran, a director of the Center for Brain and Cognition at the University of California, San Diego (UCSD), and Edward M. Hubbard, a former graduate student at UCSD and currently an assistant professor of educational psychology at the University of Wisconsin–Madison. Their test to help identify people with synesthesia relied on the Stroop effect. I had never heard of the Stroop effect, but I found out that it's named for John Ridley Stroop, a psychologist who wrote about it way back in 1935. Stroop's test was simple: He would show people the name of a color written in either that same color or in a different color. (For example, the color yellow might be written in yellow ink or in red ink.) Then he would ask them to say the name of the written word. Stroop found that it took people longer to respond when the color of the ink didn't match the name of the color.

When Dr. Ramachandran and Dr. Hubbard used this method to test synesthetes and nonsynesthetes, they found that it typically took nonsynesthetes longer to respond. Reaction times were faster for synesthetes, and much faster if the color of the ink matched the synesthetes' particular color associations for that word.

These same two doctors devised yet another simple way to test for synesthesia, this time using numbers. They created a field of 5s and inserted several 2s among them. They showed it to people and asked them to find the 2s. The researchers found that synesthetes completed the task much more quickly than nonsynesthetes. Why was it so much easier for the synesthetes? Because they saw numbers in colors, and since the 2s were a different color than the 5s, they stood out. I loved this diagnostic because it showed how synesthetes saw the hidden aspects of things just as I felt I did (although I don't have the number-and-color association).

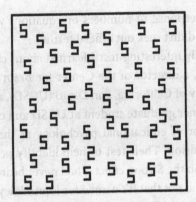

How fast can you spot the 2s?

As interesting as acquired synesthesia was, I found just as much to be fascinated by in the world of acquired savants, and I shifted my focus to this aspect of my new self. I recalled that in the television program I had seen on the savant Tammet, a psychiatrist named Darold Treffert had been featured. I did a Google search and discovered that Dr. Treffert was considered the world's leading authority on savants; some even referred to him as the dean of American savants. He'd written extensively on the subject in scientific journals, in popular media, on websites, and in his own books.

In his fifty years of practice at that point, Dr. Treffert had documented more than four hundred savant cases. Among these, he'd found only thirty cases of acquired savant syndrome. That's what I suspected I had, and I was shocked to think I might be one of only thirty people in the world to go through this.

In writing about acquired, or sudden-onset, savant syndrome, Dr. Treffert said that the ability to know or remember things that had never been learned was due to what he called genetic memory. This is knowledge that is encoded in human DNA but that remains inaccessible to most people. "The only way such embedded skills and knowledge can be there innately," Dr. Treffert claimed, "is through the genetic transfer of such knowledge and abilities.

They come 'factory installed' and remain dormant, in all of us, until tapped by some central nervous system illness or catastrophe, perhaps as a back-up system." Dr. Treffert noted that people don't question how birds instinctively know migration patterns that they have never been taught. Monarch butterflies travel to the same twenty-three-acre spot in Mexico, though it takes them three generations to do it. Why isn't it possible for humans to have innate, instinctive abilities?

Dr. Treffert wasn't the only expert to propose this theory. Far across the globe, in Australia, Allan Snyder, the director of the Centre for the Mind at the University of Sydney, had been doing research on savants since the 1990s, and he had also come to the conclusion that savant skills are innate. In a 2010 interview with *Psychology Today*, Dr. Snyder said that savants "can tap into information that exists in all our brains."

This concept made a great deal of sense to me, since I was certain that nothing I was currently thinking came from my memory. I just had not been exposed to the topics that now interested me, and I'd never learned how to do the things I could now do. The thought that this was some sort of hidden instinct, passed down through the ages, was thrilling.

What wasn't so thrilling was the fact that so many of the savants I was reading about had numerous mental challenges despite their "islands of genius," as Dr. Treffert described their extraordinary abilities. I didn't feel as disadvantaged as they were, but it did make me worry I might lose some of my normal faculties if this savant syndrome progressed somehow. I had heard the unfortunate term *idiot savant* before, and in my research I learned that it was coined in 1887 by the same man who first described the disorder we know as Down syndrome: British physician John Langdon Down. *Idiot* was not as pejorative back then, and the word *savant* came from the French word *savoir*, "to know." (Today, the constellation of symptoms is referred to as *savant syndrome;* it's best not to use the term *autistic savant,* since only about 50 percent of people with savant syndrome are autistic.) In his three decades of work at an asylum, Down identified ten people who had both significant mental challenges and remarkable skills in specific areas. The people he studied had extraordinary musical, artistic, mathematical, or mechanical skills as well as astounding memories; they were not allowed in mainstream society due to their mental deficits apart from these skills. My throat tightened as I thought about a time when people with savant syndrome were institutionalized.

The first textbook to include descriptions of savants was written in 1914 by A. F. Tredgold. It had a title that stung: *Mental Deficiency.* I found a scanned copy of the original book in an online database and pored over the yellowed pages. Tredgold dedicated the book "To all those persons of sound mind who are interested in the welfare of their less fortunate fellow-creatures," and included a chapter called "Idiot Savants." In it, he reviewed everything that had been written on the subject so far. I cringed when I read his assertion that savants weren't really idiots but rather "imbeciles or merely feeble-minded." It was painful to see people described this way. But when I read that Tredgold believed that a savant's talent must be due to "constant exercise," or practice, I knew he was dead wrong. I had never practiced any of my new talents; they just appeared. Seeing how off base he was about this aspect of savantism made it easier for me to disregard his other hurtful comments.

In all my research on savant syndrome, I've been most drawn to the stories of those people who, like me, suddenly acquired this gift. One of them was Tony Cicoria, an orthopedic surgeon from New York. In 1994, at the age of forty-two, he was using a pay phone during a rainstorm and was struck by lightning. When the bolt coursed through his body, he had the experience of being outside of himself. "I saw my own body on the ground," he told Oliver Sacks in an interview for *The New Yorker*. "I said to myself, 'Oh, shit, I'm dead.' . . . Then—slam! I was back."

Aside from feeling tired and having a few problems with memory, Dr. Cicoria was okay. Like me, he had a neurological evaluation that didn't indicate any permanent brain damage. But also like me, he found his life changing in very unexpected ways. Lucky for him, his memory problems went away. In their place, he told Sacks, "Suddenly over two or three days, there was this insatiable desire to listen to piano music." Nobody was more surprised about this new affinity for music than Cicoria. He'd never really been interested in piano music until that point. This made me think about my own newfound interest in math and fractals after a lifetime of hating math.

What's more, Dr. Cicoria soon felt it wasn't enough just to listen to the piano; he had an urge to play. He then started hearing original music in his head and had a desire to compose. So he began to study music. He still worked full-time as a surgeon and was unchanged in every other regard, but soon he was rising at 4:00 a.m. to practice, and after work, he played well into the night. It was a miraculously happy story, I thought, until I read that he and his wife divorced in 2004. When I learned that, I was so grateful that I hadn't been married before my injury. Can you imagine your spouse waking up to a stranger every day? I don't know how any of my former girlfriends would have reacted to having to sit with me, housebound, while I stared off into space pondering my visions or sat for hours doing research. I began to wonder if I'd ever find anyone who could tolerate me as I was now.

As much as that story made me reflect on the loneliness of the acquired savant, I took joy in the next several cases I studied. I particularly liked the story of Alonzo Clemons of Boulder, Colorado. As an infant, he suffered a brain injury in a fall, and though he could scarcely speak in complete sentences, Clemons could sculpt out of clay any animal he saw in uncanny detail, using no tools other than his hands. In fact, all he needed to do was glance at the animal once, and then he stored the image photographically in his mind and could complete an entirely accurate sculpture. His desire to sculpt started shortly after his head injury. As a child, he would take the shortening out of the cupboards in his family home and set to work compulsively sculpting animals; finally, someone bought him some clay. To this day, wherever he goes, he carries with him a duffle bag with several bricks of clay, just in case he sees something he has to sculpt. After reading his story, I was really glad my injury didn't rob me of the ability to communicate. I didn't choose to communicate often, but something inside me was compelled to share what I knew.

Clemons worked on his sculptures for twenty years in solitude. But when the film *Rain Man*, which was inspired by the remarkable abilities of the savant Kim Peek, came out, the public became more interested in Clemons's work. He now shows his art and has been featured on many TV shows, including *60 Minutes* and the Discovery Channel's *World of Wonder.*

Not far from Clemons, in Denver, lives another man who acquired savant abilities. Derek Amato was forty when hijinks at a backyard barbecue changed his life. Someone tossed a football near the in-ground pool, and then the game became catching the football over the water. On one toss, Amato dove into the shallow end of a pool and struck his head on the pool's floor. "I remember the impact being very loud. It was like a bomb had gone off. And I knew I hit my head hard enough that I was hurt. I knew I was hurt badly," he said in a Science Channel documentary. He felt like blood was pouring out of his ears, though it was not. He was admitted to the hospital with a serious concussion and soon noticed some memory loss and hearing loss.

A few days after the barbecue, he was released from the hospital, and he sat down at a keyboard at a friend's house and began to play. Though he'd played a little guitar, he had never played piano before, but suddenly he was a virtuoso. It was original music. And it was beautiful. He continued until about two the next morning, afraid the ability would be short-lived. He and his friend couldn't understand what was happening. "It was no 'Mary Had a Little Lamb,'" Amato said.

"As I shut my eyes, I found these black-and-white structures moving from left to right, which in fact would represent, in my mind, a fluid and continuous stream of musical notation," Amato later wrote in a blog post on the Wisconsin Medical Society's website. "I could not only play and compose, but I would later discover that I could recall a prior played piece of music as if it had been etched in my mind's eye."

In an interview on the *Today* show, Amato admitted that there were downsides to the injury. "I deal with the fluorescent-light issues," he told Matt Lauer. "I collapse sometimes out of the blue. And the migraines and the headaches are intense. And my hearing is half gone." He called the lingering symptoms "a price tag on this particular gift." When I heard him say that on the video, I thought of my own OCD, PTSD, and other problems. I agreed with him that though these issues presented a challenge, I wouldn't trade my new abilities for life without them.

Orlando Serrell is another interesting acquired savant. In 1979, when he was ten years old, he was playing baseball, and while he was making a run for first base, a baseball struck him on the left side of the head. He fell to the ground and remained there for a few moments, then got up and continued to play. "I didn't tell my parents, therefore, I had no medical treatment for the accident," he wrote on his website. He did have a headache for a long while following the incident, he said. Soon, he noticed he had developed the ability to do calendrical calculations; he could tell you the day of the week associated with any date. If you said, *March 28, 1957*, he would answer, correctly, *Thursday*. He can also tell you what the weather was and what he was doing on any given day since his accident. In 2002 he was invited by NBC's *Dateline* to undergo a brain scan at Columbia University, and he appeared in a special on savants. His case made me want to know exactly which parts of my brain had been affected by my injury.

I was glad to finally come across the case of a female with savant syndrome, as the condition is even more rare in women. According to experts, when it comes to savant syndrome, men outnumber women by about six to one. Why? Researchers are still trying to figure it out, but some theories suggest that it may have something to do with the way the brain develops in the womb. Also, the savant syndrome is often associated with autism, and autism is more common in males.

The lone female savant I came across was a child named Nadia. In the 1970s, she drew beautiful pictures of horses, and her drawings were so fine they were compared to those of Rembrandt and Leonardo da Vinci. But she lost her drawing abilities when she learned to speak, according to the British psychologist Lorna Selfe.

I cobbled together what I was learning about acquired synesthesia and savantism to get a better picture of what was going on in my own mind. The stories of people with such gifts were comforting to me, though I hadn't yet come across anyone with what I suspected I had, both acquired synesthesia and acquired savantism. The experiences of savants and synesthetes still didn't explain what was happening in my life. Even Tammet had had what I considered the good fortune to be born the way he was. I doubted he could truly relate to my conflicted feelings about my new identity. My alternating shock and euphoria about the emergence of my new sensory perceptions added a layer to the experience I'm not sure people who've had synesthesia or savant syndrome their whole lives can imagine. Would I ever feel at home in my own skin and have that sort of acceptance and grace about my abilities?

Though I looked to Tammet and other fellow synesthetes and savants with extraordinary gifts for clues and guidance, I was left with the feeling I would have to forge my own path.

CHAPTER SEVEN

The Edge of a Circle

I N MY ISOLATION, I felt the profound change of the shape of my own world. My life used to be a mile wide and an inch deep: I covered a lot of ground running around, but I barely scratched the surface of things with my superficial pursuits. Now, it was an inch wide and a mile deep. I was practically immobile, working from my spot at the computer most days. I focused on the tiniest thing and pondered it incessantly, plumbing this narrow but very deep space.

It was during this time of major shifts in my perception — started by my trauma and made greater by this silent laboratory of sorts — that I found my intellectual passion. I became fascinated with pi, that irrational, infinite number that corresponds to a circle's circumference divided by its diameter. To me, that irrational number became a fundamental building block of everything around me, a signifier of nature's perfect symmetry, repeated over and over throughout our world. I saw it everywhere I looked with my new brain: in light reflected off glass, in the corona of a street lamp, even in the virtual scaffolding of a rainbow.

My fascination with pi began in 2005. On a rare foray outside, I noticed the light bouncing off a car window in the form of an arc, and the concept came to life. Like most visual phenomena now, it was hardly just light bouncing off glass but an extraordinary geometric display: a ball of light was where the beam hit the glass. Rays fanned out from it like the spokes of an illuminated bicycle wheel or the radii of a circle. They were iridescent and I was rapt and lost in the potential infinity of it all. It looked like a laser light show my favorite bar might have put on in the old days, only a million times better. Staring at the display, I felt an overwhelming sense of stimulation and inspiration. To the new me, so entranced by math and physics for the first time, it was a revelation.

I was literally fist-pumping and saying, "Oh my God! This is amazing!" over and over that day when I first understood that what I was seeing was a representation of pi. It clicked for me because the circle I saw was subdivided by the light rays and I realized each ray was really a representation of the radius dividing the circle into pieces. I realized that if I added up the areas of all these pieces, which were sort of like slices of a cake, they would equal the circle's area. Measuring that value would be a much easier way to figure out the value of pi than the difficult "circumference of a circle divided by its diameter" method I had once struggled to understand in school. In my Internet searches about circles and diameters and radii, I had learned that pi was a confounding problem because the circumference divided by the diameter was irrational: rather than corresponding to a clean fraction, the number stretched out to infinity in decimal form, with no repeating pattern. If you divide 1 by 3, you get 0.33333333, with 3s repeating forever. Divide 1 by 7 and you get the infinitely repeating pattern 0.142857142857142857. Divide a circle's circumference by its diameter and you get a number that begins 3.14159265358 and just keeps going. Mathematicians are still calculating new digits of pi, out into the quadrillions, and no one has yet found a real repeating pattern. No wonder it had always been so hard to understand.

Part of the trouble is that no one has a way to accurately measure the circumference or area of a perfect circle. Instead, mathematicians have to approximate. One way of calculating the value of pi dates back to the Greek mathematician Archimedes. Around 250 BC, he tried to find the area of a circle by placing one polygon inside a circle and another polygon outside the circle. He calculated the perimeter of the two polygons and theorized that the value of pi lay between those two numbers. Then he kept increasing the number of sides of the polygons — working his way up to ninety-six sides — so the areas of the two polygons got closer to equaling each other. Using this method, he calculated that the value of pi was between $3 \frac{10}{71}$ and $3 \frac{1}{7}$. The ancient Greeks didn't use decimals, but his fractions were the equivalent of about 3.1408 and 3.1429, respectively — not too far off the figure we use today.

I had never been taught about Archimedes or this visual approach, but now that I had arrived at the realization independently, I wanted to run through the streets announcing my profound discovery. I wanted to tell everyone this was a great secret revealed. Suddenly an idea I'd known in school only as "that 3.14 number" took on a relevance it had never had for me in a textbook or lecture.

I raced home and began my research further into pi that very day. As I read academic papers and popular-science articles online, I started to feel that pi literally defined everything — not just the ratios in a circle, but all of creation. It pertained to so many naturally occurring spheres, from pebbles to planets. And in more complex mathematics, like calculus, it helped define slope. I thought about the spirals of my seashell and draining water and coffee swirls. My own pupils were circles. Where would we be without the invention of the wheel? Circles were everywhere I looked and they felt fundamental to existence.

I began trying to describe what I saw to the rare visitor or person who telephoned. I said things like "Have you ever seen those boats where you push the lever forward from stop to fast? Push that lever all the way up and think of it as an obtuse, greater-than-ninety-degree angle, say a hundred-and-seventy-nine-degree angle, a really large one. Move that lever back down to a right angle, then slowly bring it down to an acute, less-than-ninety-degree angle until you collapse it in on itself. Think that every click along that lever makes a certain triangle. And every triangle is defined by pi at a certain value." While this visual helped me a great deal and seemed very on point, my audience remained confused.

I wished I could give everyone the eureka moment I had had that day with the car—a circle subdivided by glistening, illuminated triangles. But when I tried to describe my inspiration, people told me that it would have been just an arc of light or a halo or a reflection to them. I couldn't believe it was so mundane to them when for me it was a peak experience. I searched for the words to best represent this. I would wave my hands in the air, tracing what I'd seen with a pointed finger. All I got in return were blank stares. I realized that things would never be the same for me—all my life I would see down deep into the structure of things while everyone I knew was still skating on the surface. It was as though I'd been fitted with some sort of microscopic, x-ray-vision contact lenses. I searched for the words to capture its beauty and, more than that, the truth I believed its structure represented, but I was stammering.

Finally, I picked up a pencil and tried to sketch it.

I had never been able to draw in the past, but I was now pretty adept. The pencil didn't feel like a foreign object in my hand but an extension of me and my mind. I felt compelled to draw and did almost nothing else. I found I was better able to represent things on paper than I had been. The joke in my family until now had been that when we played Pictionary, my doodles were always the worst! For one round of the game in which I had to represent the god Zeus, my scratch marks were little more than a carrot shape for a mountain and a zigzag for a lightning bolt above it.

I was amazed by my sudden facility with a pencil. It was as though someone else were clutching my fist and guiding my hand. This was another ability I'd never had before, and I had to set the pencil down for a moment to take it all in. What really made it come together, however, was when, in a rare conversation during my continued self-imposed isolation, a friend suggested that I add a ruler and a compass to my toolbox. I began to draw forms very close to the beauty I'd witnessed.

When I first tried to render the vision, I drew a perfect circle with a smooth perimeter, which was *not* what I had seen. The circle I saw was not perfectly curved — the circumference of it was jagged. It was more of a polygon with countless sides and filled with triangles, only approximating a perfect circle. So, as I drafted circle after circle at my desk, I began filling them with triangles. As I added more triangles I realized I was filling in more and more area at the circle's edge.

"You can only fill in more and more triangles," I said to my mom during one late-night phone call about this quest.

"Hence, pi goes to infinity," she responded.

Her statement made everything click, and I realized how this insight was reflected in the circles I saw all around me and had been attempting to draw. What if the base of these triangles became smaller and smaller? First I filled a circle with 60 triangles, then 180:

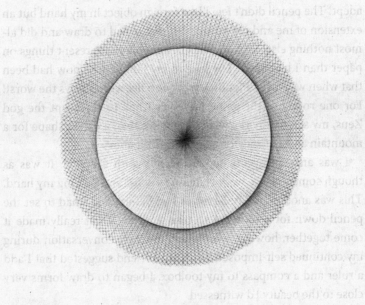

Then 360:

All the way up to 720, when the width of the pencil's lead wouldn't allow for any more lines:

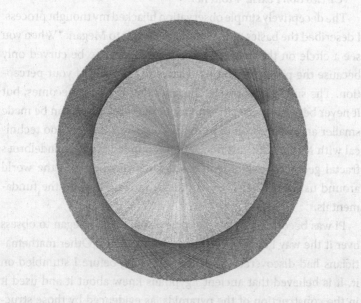

One day my daughter, Megan, was halfway through an episode of *Pokémon* when she hollered a question to me: "Dad, how does the TV work?" I explained that each image is made up of hundreds of little rectangular pixels, and when the pixels change color, they change the larger picture too. Just then a commercial for Overstock.com, with its giant *O* logo, came on, and Megan said, "That's *impossible*, Dad. How do you make a circle out of rectangles?"

It was like a bomb went off in my mind. In a matter of minutes, I was no longer just a receiver of geometric imagery or a researcher; I was a theorist.

Ever since the mugging, curved objects in my line of sight had lost their smooth edges. They looked jagged and inexplicably discrete from their surroundings, and while I had spent years puzzling over the distortion, its significance had eluded me, and my drawings hadn't cracked the code. That afternoon I found the right words.

"Circles don't exist," I told her.

The deceptively simple observation hijacked my thought process. I described the basics of the familiar concept to Megan: "When you see a circle on the television, the edges appear to be curved only because the pixels are so tiny relative to the scale of your perception. The smaller the pixels, the smoother the edge becomes, but it never becomes perfectly smooth because the pixels can be made smaller and smaller, on to infinity." I didn't want to get too technical with Megan, but this realization reminded me of Mandelbrot's fractal geometry, which emphasized the roughness in the world around us. In my head, I was quickly moving beyond the fundamentals.

Pi was becoming my mathematical soul mate. I began to obsess over it the way I did the cleanliness of my hands. Other mathematicians had discovered the utility of pi long before I stumbled on it. It is believed that ancient Egyptians knew about it and used it in the construction of the pyramids, as evidenced by those structures' proportions. Pi has even been found in the Mandelbrot set. Its value lay in mathematics — not just in geometry but also in calculus applications and computing algorithms. The record for calculating pi (as of this writing) — which has been an obsession of people around the world ever since pi was first discovered — was achieved in March 2013 by Ed Karrels of Santa Clara University, in California. He computed the number to eight quadrillion places using a supercomputer. Though the sophisticated calculations of pi humbled me, I realized all of us were seeking the same thing.

However, I thought even the most sophisticated attempts to calculate pi were not taking it down to the quantum level — not one that I was able to find from my humble home computer station, anyway. So I began contemplating a hypothetical correction using one of the concepts for which Max Planck was awarded the Nobel

Prize: the Planck length, an infinitesimally small unit of measurement equal to 1.62 x 10^{-35} meters. Just to clarify, that's millions, billions, trillions, and even quadrillions times smaller than anything that can be seen with the naked eye. The Planck length is the scale of length measurement where the usual rules of gravity break down and quantum mechanics comes into play. It's also the smallest possible building block of space in the universe that can be observed (or exist relative to us). If the triangles I placed in my circle were each on the scale of a Planck length — *would that not be a more perfect pi?* I later posted my theory about this on a physics forum online because I was so sure I was the first to discover it.

I didn't know much about academic procedures and I was far from being able to write a journal article on my thoughts and submit it for peer review, but this little step in taking my thoughts public was a real change for me. I found that society interested me again — if only in the context of having a conversation with people about math. I had some great responses, which encouraged me, and some real trolls, who insulted me and made me realize online forums aren't the best place to seek feedback. But it was still a big step for me to post my thoughts.

After that brief and mixed-results excursion into public discourse, I doubled up on my reading and ignored the pull of the outside world. Historically speaking, I was in good company — Archimedes was allegedly so engrossed in pi that he failed to notice when Roman soldiers captured his home city of Syracuse. Before he was beheaded, he yelled, "Don't disturb my circles!" I understood how he felt.

The term *pi*, which is the sixteenth letter of the Greek alphabet, was first used to describe the irrational number in a 1706 paper by the mathematician William Jones. The concept of pi has existed for four thousand years, and it can be used as a litmus test to indicate where humans were technologically at any given time. As Petr Beckmann wrote in *A History of π*, "The history of π is a quaint little mirror of the history of man." I read that Simon Newcomb, the astronomer and mathematician who accurately measured the speed of light in the nineteenth century, had been quoted as saying humankind's fascination with pi vastly transcends practical need. "Ten decimals are sufficient to give the circumference of the earth to the fraction of an inch," he said, "and thirty decimals would give the circumference of the whole visible universe to a quantity imperceptible with the most powerful telescope." But as humankind advanced, so did the utility of pi. Since ancient times, it has been important in construction and architecture. Now, everything from manufacturing machine parts to navigation and global positioning makes use of the constant in engineering formulas. Its infinite trail stretches out before us like a road map to the future, driving us forward. If pi really is tied to the Planck length, I imagine this finding could prove even more useful, for everything from space travel to supercomputing to things we have not yet imagined. If explorers from another world one day found our lifeless planet and excavated the ruins, I fantasized they would conclude, "Throughout their history, humans sought the end of pi."

Realizing this made me want to perfect pi — to get it to the closest possible measurement of all. I went deeper within myself than I ever had before to attempt this. I became a virtual hermit as I pursued my study of pi. I knew I was obsessed. However, I had read that obsession was key to savants' capabilities and supposed this was how I was going to be from now on. I didn't try to change my behavior. I was growing to like the new me.

Even in the beginning of my pi quest, when I was energized by my newfound artistic abilities, I understood the contradictions in my behavior. I was creatively extroverted — practically evangelistic about my visions, in fact — but physically introverted and still flinching at the sound of footsteps. I rarely felt up to tackling my fear, but my daughter, Megan, inspired me to try. Early one eve-

ning in 2005, I noticed that my seven-year-old was staying cooped
up in the living room with her friend Dylan rather than playing
outdoors. My fear for my own safety extended to my precious
child, and I never even let her go out into the yard. It occurred to
me that she was feeling the same isolation I'd created for myself. I
dug out my telescope from the closet and shouted from the entry-
way:

"C'mon, guys, we're going outside to look at the stars."

"Are you sure, Daddy?" Megan was surprised to see me even approach the front door.

"Absolutely; come on."

I was almost finished setting up the tripod outside when my
neighbor from two doors down approached.

"Excuse me, you're stepping on my irises," she said.

"That's a good joke!" I responded, thinking she was referring to
the irises of her eyes and the high-powered lens of the telescope.
I was becoming really good at reading body language and having
empathy, but verbal cues were not my strong suit.

"It's not a joke. You're in my flower bed!"

"Oh, I'm sorry . . . I'll move down five feet or so. I live right there."

"What do you mean, you live right there? No one lives there," the
woman said, sweeping her hand toward my house. The roof was
partially caved in — due to a fallen tree branch — and pigeons were
flying in and out of the attic.

"No, really, I've lived here for the last six years," I replied. The
neighbor walked back home, incredulous.

My time outside my house was brief; I was pulled back in to my
studies of pi. My isolation reinforced by my obsession with this
number, I continued to learn its history and practice drawing my
visions and equations by hand. I began to lose all sense of time and
found myself practically hypnotized by the pursuit. I concluded
that when scientists used computers to illustrate a formula, they

forfeited the opportunity to witness each individual step, and much of the information about the underlying math and how it actually worked was lost. I may not have been a mathematician, but not a step was lost on me in my geometric bunker.

I almost didn't remember the old barhopping, good-time Jason now as I hunched over my drawing tablet or sat for hours in front of the computer, soaking up all that I'd missed during my formal education and chasing pi's infinite trail out into space. I began to take solace in my isolation because I had found my passion, my constant companion: my research.

After pi revealed itself to me in a way that could be drawn, the other images came to me, one after another. The floodgates opened and I could finally express what was going on in my newly fertile mind. I could see geometric representations for equations related to relativity, for example, and to the photon double-slit experiment and to particle fusion and to the way prime numbers live for me at vectors within a sphere. Nothing was a simple equation; it had to have form.

I bought several artist's drawing tablets and boxes of new pencils and spent every moment — at the breakfast table or my desk — working on putting these visions on paper.

One of the earliest things I did was plot the way I saw prime numbers: out in space, in front of me. I drew a circle and began filling it with sequential, boxed numbers, setting off the primes by coloring in their spaces with a red or blue pencil. Instead of tracing this in the air while trying to describe it verbally, I could show people something concrete about what I was thinking. Though it was still unusual for me to see people, on those occasions when I did, I found them nodding at my explanations. Even if they didn't understand it completely, most said it was beautiful and had an interesting pattern.*

---

*Some of the dates on the following illustrations are later than this time because I

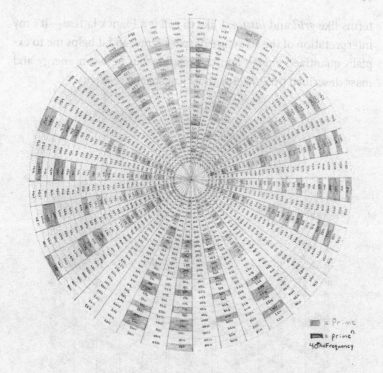

My synesthetic visions were solved and unsolved, explaining mathematical concepts to me but not explained *by* mathematical concepts (at least, none that I was aware of). I began to think of them as a different way into known concepts, as though I were seeing math from a fresh angle. To me, they were so provocative that they made things relevant for the first time in my life and made me want to know about the realm they came from.

I also tried my hand at a shape that artists, mathematicians, physicists, and others have been drawing for thousands of years. Some describe it as sacred geometry, while others use scientific

continually worked to perfect them over several years. I present the best of the updated renderings here.

terms like *grid* and *lattice*. I like to call it a Planck lattice — it's my interpretation of the structure of space-time, and it helps me to explain quantized energy and the relationship between energy and mass described by Einstein's theory of special relativity.

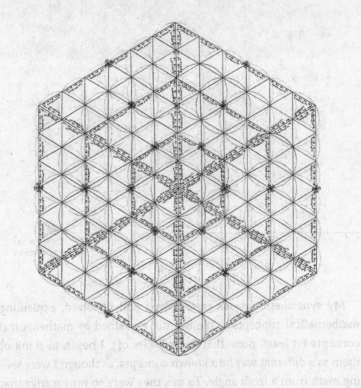

Each side of every small equilateral triangle in this diagram represents a Planck length. I started with a single point and drew triangles outward until a lattice appeared. I realized that every point in space-time needed to be one or whole multiples of the Planck length away from all the others. This requirement, in my opinion, automatically creates the gridlike structure of space-time that Albert Einstein described.

Another theme that inspired me to draw was the idea of wave-particle duality, a concept introduced by Einstein in 1905. He had previously described light as made of photons. However, he knew that light sometimes acted like a wave instead of a stream of particles. I wanted to capture that moment of transition, when light is both particle and wave. This is what I saw in my mind when I imagined it. I also saw this in my mind's eye when thinking about parallel universes. I realized there were so many discrete numbers of places you could be, and each one of those had a certain probability. A photon can follow all possible paths, just as the center point of this drawing could. This image arises in my imagination now whenever I think of probability, even when I'm making mundane decisions about which actions to take during an ordinary day.

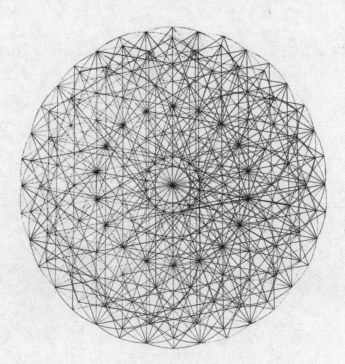

It occurred to me that not only did light move as waves or particles across the space-time grid, so did I — what little I moved those days. I spent many hours absorbed in translating my ideas into drawings from that point onward. The artwork allowed me to express my rich new inner life. It also gave me a sense of connectedness, in that I was now at least reading about other people and trying to take part in a conversation, even if my continuing fear of face-to-face human contact kept me from leaving the house. In so many ways, my art was saving me.

CHAPTER EIGHT

Inflection Point

DRAWINGS OF MY visions and ideas were now piled high all around me in every room. I was drifting off to sleep in front of the TV one late April night in 2006 when a local news bulletin startled me into a raw, uncomfortable consciousness. The anchor reported that a human skeleton had been found over the weekend by two young boys cutting trails in the woods, and I recognized the location as a stretch of evergreens only one hundred dred yards from my brother's front door. After all this time, could it be possible that the answer to my brother's disappearance had been that close?

I dialed the station's hot line, and the switchboard forwarded my call to the police department in Kent, a town near where my brother had lived at the time of his disappearance. I told the receptionist what my brother was wearing the night he disappeared — an Alaska Helicopters Inc. jacket and a Los Angeles Raiders baseball cap — and after an excruciating silence, she confirmed that this description matched the clothes discovered with the remains. Before the news even sank in, I phoned my mother and father, one right after the other. They cried into their receivers.

The mystery of my brother's vanishing was both solved and unsolved; I learned that a garrote was found next to the body and that the hyoid bone was missing from John's neck, consistent with strangling, but the police investigation was inconclusive. With no active criminal investigation going on, the specter of suicide hung over my family, though I refused to believe it. The uncertainty was more comfortable than the conclusion, and after all, I'd learned to coexist with the inexplicable.

I accompanied my mom to identify the remains. It was so hard to see my brother reduced to skeleton form. I stared for a long time at the contours of his skull and recognized it as very similar to my own; now that I'd grown so thin, I could see my bone structure when looking in the mirror. The similarities in the outlines and the angles were stunning to me. I tried to focus on that geometry instead of the horror before me.

John's death made me realize how far I'd drifted from my family. Perhaps it was time to reconnect. Though I'd felt renewed kinship with my parents over our mutual loss of John, I still couldn't bring myself to reach out to them beyond our initial coming-together for the funeral. I couldn't break my isolation.

My brother's death only reinforced my fear of the outside world and assured me that I was on the right side of my walls, where I remained. It had been three and a half years since I first retreated into the dark refuge of my home. Months of quiet study followed my brother's death, during which memories of him interrupted my thoughts regularly.

Some of the memories were bittersweet. One summer day when I was about nine and John was eleven, we were in the Alaska woods and a car came tearing through a dirt road toward us, kicking up a huge cloud of dust. We had already made dozens of dead-end trails in the forest around the cabin, fitting the paths with tripwires made of fishing line and digging half-foot holes in the ground that were camouflaged with leaves to trap any bad guys who might approach. John hurriedly shaved the leaves off a six-foot fireweed to fashion a spear and launched it at the car, which came screeching to a halt. Out came one very angry, very drunk lumberjack. We boys ran like hell down one of our trails, dissolving into fits of giggles when the tree cutter fell like an oak himself, tripped by one of our wires. Then he got up and got close enough to grab John by the ankle. He screamed at us for some time but eventually returned to his car. We high-fived each other and celebrated our ability to protect ourselves; the trap had worked, on the whole. We thought we were immortal at that moment, totally unaware of the dangers that awaited us in the future.

My mom married a man named Bob and we eventually moved out of our cabin to a gigantic wooden home in the wilderness in the town of Girdwood. The home was built on ten-foot stilts due to the depth of the snow. We would go through about twenty cords of wood each season there — we would split and stack them ourselves. The road nearest the town is considered the most dangerous in the state of Alaska, and it's also one of the most important routes for commerce and defense: the Seward Highway. The road goes through a national forest, continues for about five miles to our former hometown, and then passes through Chugach State Park for ten miles. After that, it goes through the skiing village of Bird and the village of Indian, and then it reenters the forest. Finally, it passes along the Gulf of Alaska and has vistas so stunning they are fatally distracting. Collisions there are almost always head-on.

My best memory of the house was hiding up in my loft, enjoying the sound of rain on the roof or feeling the awe of the sound of snow sliding off it and down to the ground. First you would hear *crack!* Then: *whoosh!* Then: *boom! Boom!* and as many booms as it took to get all the large chunks of snow off the slope at the top of the house.

Living in the wilderness proved to be too boring for John; he was so bored, he decided to call in a false fire alarm one day. I admit I aided him in that foolishness. When he handed me the phone after calling in the fire, I whimpered, "Help!" The operator sent emergency vehicles in a flash over treacherous terrain, only to find us cowering and already feeling guilty about what we'd done.

But there had once been a real fire at our place. We had carelessly thrown a bunch of newspapers we'd used to catch paint drippings into the fireplace, and they ignited the twenty-foot chimney. My mom, Toni, is now a frail lady, owing to the losses in our lives, but back in the day, you could give her an emergency and watch some sort of superhero reserve come into play. She's still remarkable and I seek her advice a lot. I remember her evacuating us and simultaneously fighting the fire with an extinguisher, getting us to safety and saving the house in the process.

I remembered the time a bully in our town began riding his motorbike up our driveway really aggressively, harassing us with countless revs of his engine just under our windows. John had no problem when I dug a trench in the road out in front of our house and filled it with gasoline and put in a fuse. I waited to hear the sound of the approaching speed demon, and as soon as I did, I set it ablaze. He came screeching to a halt in front of the wall of flames and never bothered us again. Sometimes I laughed to myself through tears at these memories. I had been a survivor at a very young age.

And then my time in Alaska ended. Our father called to ask if John and I would like to visit him in his new home in Seattle. I said yes. For some reason, John said no. When I reflect on it now, I think the divorce must have been more disturbing to John than it was to me. He was older and more aware of events, and in the way that firstborns often bear the brunt of things in a family, he took everything much harder than I did.

My plane approached Seattle, and the Space Needle might as well have been a giant exclamation point. I couldn't believe the city, with its perfect balance of nature and development: the wide expanses of the blue sound, the glittering new buildings of downtown, all interspersed with green spaces. I'd been living in the woods, after all. At the summer's end, my father and his new girlfriend, Pam, asked me if I wanted to stay and go to school there. I didn't hesitate to say yes. That was the beginning of something wonderful and new for me — a second chance in a way — but it was also the beginning of a rift between me and my brother.

Later, John did move to Seattle, but he was different, and things were never the same between us. John would like a girl, and she would like me better; we'd play a board game and I would win; I made friends more easily; and Pam chose me as her favorite. And worse, I was blissfully unaware there were hard feelings until I was about sixteen. By then John was exhibiting signs of bipolar disorder, though we didn't know what it was at the time.

What we were aware of was that John had withdrawn deep inside himself. He was distrustful of people and developed an abiding interest in animals, almost as a substitute. He would walk around in a trench coat filled with martial-arts weapons and sugar gliders, these tiny rodent pets he kept with him all the time. He always had the right leg of his pants rolled up to the knee — even in cold weather — to display a tattoo he'd gotten: a ferret in an attack position, standing on its hind legs. He grew violent. More than once, I had to pretend to pass out when he had me in a chokehold, to get him off me. John fought violently with Pam.

I began remarking to friends that my brother was becoming the most bizarre person I'd ever met. Most of them dismissed it and said, "Oh, I know someone like that too," until they actually met John and decided he topped them all.

John did get it together for a time, and he joined the navy. But when he got out, things went bad again. He became friends with a crowd of martial-arts-trained, very sexy women. Despite John's strange behavior, women liked him; he was very good-looking and quite athletic. One of these women, Keri, was his favorite, and he fathered a child with her. But there was a rival for her love, and this man reportedly threatened John on more than one occasion.

In those first months after the mugging, while I holed up in my house, I spent a lot of my time thinking about our lives. One of the women my father had married after Pam secretly beat us when he wasn't home. I coined a term for the behavior of some of my step-parents: *kill-the-cub syndrome*. When lions and other animals take mates, they often kill the offspring from their new mates' previous couplings, and I felt like those ill-fated little cubs, stuck in the mating cycle of human animals.

John and I finally spoke up about the secret beatings, and we came home from school the next day to find a truck in front of our home and a crew of movers getting our stepmom's stuff out. At that point, telling my father what had happened was all it took to get him to respond to us. He grew lonely in middle age, however, and made another bad choice. The beautiful younger woman he fell in love with had a crack-cocaine problem. He knew this when he moved her into our home. She stole a gold ring from my room as well as checks out of my checkbook. I figured this out when a check I wrote bounced and I realized the two before it were missing. I confronted her about it and she admitted she'd stolen money from my account, saying, "I did something stupid."

"You know you shouldn't leave stuff like that lying around" was all my dad would say. I was so grateful when they finally broke up and she moved out. Instrumental in that breakup was my current stepmom, Helen. She was working for my dad at the time, and with a lot of patience and love, she convinced him he could find someone better; namely, her. They've been married for some twenty years now and have a large family of stepchildren and stepgrandchildren.

Things at Mom's place weren't much better when we spent time there. She divorced again and married a Canadian man named Bill. He hit me so hard one time that my back hurt for two days.

All of these experiences did damage to John's already fragile psyche. At some point he changed from being a playmate and co-conspirator to being a menace, even to me.

He convinced me one day that a man up the street had stolen the 1967 rally sport hubcaps off his new car. It was true that the Corvette a couple of driveways up did have the same accessories my brother had lost to a thief. John ordered me to sneak over there and remove them. I was more afraid of my brother than of whoever owned that Corvette. I was only fourteen; John was sixteen. As I didn't have a growth spurt until my late teens, I was under five feet tall and only ninety pounds at that point. I went to get the hubcaps.

I approached the house stealthily and leaned down next to the sports car. I was just getting a bolt off one of the tires when a man came out swinging. He hit my face so hard that my eyes were blackened and I had to pull my lips away from my braces. When I explained to him the same tires had gone missing from my brother's car, he told me he had just picked his own car up from the dealership and the similar make of the hubcaps was only a coincidence. My brother mocked me when I returned, beaten, and admitted that he knew the man hadn't stolen them but he wanted them anyway.

During my period of reflection in the wake of the discovery of my brother's body, I worried for several weeks about whether the mental illness that might have afflicted John was actually what was wrong with me. Maybe I was just hallucinating all the stuff going on in my brain and body. John had always been so different from me that I never worried about my mental health this way. I tried to reassure myself that my behavior was still quite different from John's. And my cognitive abilities were still growing, not degenerating. The fact that these visions and thoughts were due to a remarkable change in my brain and were actually new gifts would be borne out by scientific testing one day, but at the time, I occasionally worried that I had the same devastating disease as my brother.

It was, in the end, my stomach that came to my rescue. One afternoon four years into my solitude, a simple craving inspired me to break my seclusion. My heart was set on a roast beef sandwich from Subway, located in the Tacoma Mall food court. I opened my front door for the first time in six weeks, squinting in the sunlight and clutching my entire portfolio of drawings to my chest. My greatest concern was that someone would break into my house and steal my work while I was away. The sight of my own pale skin in the sideview mirror distracted me every time I changed lanes, but I made it to the mall without incident. A few minutes after I sat down to lunch, a balding man wearing glasses eating at the next table over leaned in and asked about my illustrations.

Evangelistic as ever, I launched into a spirited retelling of my story and did my best to explain what each of my drawings represented. The man—whose name I never learned—was stunned. He introduced himself simply as a physicist from a local university and said to me, "You don't have the vocabulary yet because you haven't been studying in a formal setting, but you understand some pretty complicated concepts. If you can, you really should go back to school."

Somewhere in my brain, a switch was flipped. Half an hour later, I took the first, miraculous step toward recovery. I drove to Tacoma Community College to sign up for some classes. I found a professor in the math department's office who told me the current semester had started a week earlier and registration was now closed, but seeing my determination, she relented and gave me a quiz to take home over the weekend. If I passed, she'd let me in.

I worked day and night on my ticket back to civilization. I scored a perfect 100 and started classes the following Monday.

CHAPTER NINE

Joe College

THE WEEKEND BEFORE I started classes, I took the blankets off my windows. Sunlight flooded the interior of my home and I caught a glimpse of myself in the living-room mirror. Though the image didn't change my new, hopeful mood, I realized I looked pretty frail. I used to spend hours on tanning beds, bronzing my skin to better show off my muscles. Now, my arms were thin as rails, and I was as white as a ghost. I decided to make an appointment with my doctor for a checkup in preparation for starting school. He drew some blood. He called me later and was very concerned — I had the lowest vitamin D level he'd ever seen. Four years of self-imposed exile had taken their toll. The doctor prescribed a weekly megadose of the vitamin to take orally. The pharmacist took a look at the scrip and asked if there'd been some mistake. I encouraged him to call the doctor, which he did; the dose was correct. I took my first pill the morning I got ready for my first day of school. I was taking two classes: chemistry and math.

I looked out the window that Monday morning, and I felt as though I were watching the sunrise for the first time in my life. It was the most beautiful daybreak I had ever seen. The sky was pink and orange and there were clouds of the deepest indigo streaking through the sherbet-colored air. My vitamin D deficiency reminded me how long it had been since I'd spent any time in daylight. What else had I missed these past four years? I wondered. I decided before I went to school I'd head out and take some pictures of the sky. As I walked toward the east, pointing my camera here and there to get the most of the sunrise, early-morning commuters looked at me curiously and then up at the sky. They must have thought they were missing some rare celestial event, because it was only a sunrise, their glances seemed to say. How could they be immune to this? I wondered. It was the most glorious beginning of a very important morning — truly a new dawn.

I stuffed my textbooks into a rolling suitcase and tucked my prized drawings under my arm and made my way to the beginning course of the Introductory Math series at Tacoma Community College. As I walked through the throngs of people on campus, I felt, for some reason, like I was coming home. After spending the entirety of my twenties in a perpetual bar crawl, I was now surrounded by (mostly) serious, studious adults for the first time in my life. I felt a little self-conscious because I noticed that, at thirty-five, I was more than a decade older than most of the other students, but I was really excited.

I knew I'd gone there to study math, but what it felt like was a foreign-language immersion course. My previous "school of life" education was five days a week in the nine-to-five world and seven nights a week in the social world, and I was never at a loss for words. But now I needed the *right* words — a new set of tools to better express myself and all the new thoughts I was having. I remembered the observation the physicist had made that inspired me to go back to school: he'd said I needed to acquire the vocabulary to explain myself. Instead of just *drawing* what I saw, I had to learn how to explain it and become fluent in the language of math as well as the everyday language of research.

The minute I stepped onto campus, I heard snippets of conversation from the students and faculty walking by. I listened carefully, hoping to catch these precious, new words like fish in my net. I trawled for them even there on the walkways and hoped they would help my tongue catch up to my racing mind. I fantasized for a moment about the day I could have a smooth, satisfying conversation about math without stopping every other sentence, struggling to explain what I meant without the associated accepted theories to back it up and the proper vocabulary to express it. Words are powerful and illuminate so much when you have the right ones at your disposal. My words then were wrong and lacking in specificity. I relied on long-drawn-out explanations of my ideas, and I'd never seen anyone react with the bright light of understanding in his eyes that I saw when I drew it for someone. When I got frustrated, I would just blurt out, "Let me draw it for you." I felt like an immigrant to a foreign land where people spoke a different language. I was so new to it all. I wanted to become one of them, a citizen of my new land.

But first I had to make it past the men mowing the lawn on campus. Seeing them stopped me in my tracks. I was fascinated by the angles of the mowers, how they changed as the ground's slope changed. I thought about the blades of grass, and then my mind automatically cut everything around the area into slices of the grid structure of space-time as I saw it — all webby, with lines extending as far as I could see. I saw these strange little fuzzy moving particles everywhere on the grid; more in some areas and less in others. I paused for a moment, as I was not sure why the air was so filled with those particles. I noticed the strong, sweet aroma of cut grass as I saw the particles in that magnified grid, and then I finally realized they were the pieces of cut grass floating through the air. It's interesting to me how that happened, how I was momentarily lost. When I focus on something, it's as though my mind is a camera and that camera switches to autofocus and zooms in. It's not something I can control and I don't always know how the tiny patterns I see at this level translate to the environment around me. I lose perspective. Have you ever seen a bird on the branch of a tree in the distance and wanted to capture it with your camera? Then you zoom in and it's just a jumble of branches and you have to search around for the bird with your new focus. This is what my brain is like.

My zoom lens then pulled back so I saw things as they were and gained the perspective I needed to keep walking through this plane. I saw the particles swirl and imagined the tiniest of them going up my nose. This startled me, as I'm allergic to grass, and I tried not to panic. My brain switched to a sort of computational mode as it looked at this large, vivid grid pattern with the grass swirls. I determined the path with the fewest grass particles and walked through it like a maze.

Though I'd managed to map out a path to class, I was distracted yet again when I noticed the geometry of the plants along the way. The way the leaves and blossoms fanned out, the leaves or petals subdividing a circle with multiples — say, four leaves or eight petals — sent my mind into overdrive as it tried to calculate the geometry of flowers. It occurred to me that the number of petals or leaves in a group was seldom a prime number. And then I started thinking about how that number of petals or leaves might be an evolutionary advantage in terms of how the plants used light and space; perhaps that arrangement made the most efficient use of the space-time grid and better captured light for photosynthesis.

I hadn't been outdoors in daylight for such a long time that I was seeing nearly everything around me with new eyes. It was all I could do to keep walking to class. The great beauty of nature's mathematical truths was all around me, and I realized that I was experiencing the reality of living mathematics, whereas most people saw only its map and then confused the map with the actual territory and got misled. I knew that mathematicians described nature with their formulas. But to me, there was something deeper than that going on. I thought there was more to the nature of the universe than equations — I thought perhaps the universe spoke in its own form of math. And that math was geometry. Equations were symbolic; numbers were symbolic. But to me, geometry was *real*.

Being outdoors and looking so closely at everything made me aware of the microscopic world, and the campus struck me as a giant petri dish crawling with bacteria. There were so many people, and I was certain that they carried countless germs. I was also feeling assaulted by the cars going by on campus, the exhaust spewing from them. I'd been cloistered for so long that I'd almost forgotten cars had exhaust. I made my way to the building where my first class was and was similarly affronted by the smokers huddled by the stairs at the entrance. I walked to their extreme left, hugging the railing as I climbed the steps, and I held my breath the entire time. I was concentrating so hard on not breathing that I inadvertently touched the railing. My hand felt warm and I was overpowered by a gross feeling of filth. I found a restroom to wash up before continuing on.

Though it was really cool to see the world in such great detail, the result was that I felt quite overwhelmed and exhausted before I even got to the classroom. There was so much to keep track of — the grass particles, the petals, the bits of interesting conversation, the clustered smokers, the spewing exhaust pipes, the potential lurking germs. I mapped them all out in my mind and found it hard to snap out of thinking about each obsessively. That promised land, that campus of my dreams, was also for me a forest with many hazards.

I stumbled down the hallway with my book bag, opening the

doors with my feet or my elbows to avoid touching the handles with their millions of microbes. As terrified and overstimulated as I felt, I made a promise to myself that day that I would not drop out. I began to think of ways to avoid letting my discomfort with germs stop me from reaching my goals.

From then on, I brought a large number of hand wipes to school with me. In every classroom, I zipped open my rolling suitcase and took out a handful of wipes to sterilize my desk and chair before sitting down. The few students who shot me dubious looks as I did that got treated to the sight of a grimy, blackened cloth. They lost their skepticism with a chorus of "Ewww!" and some of them even introduced themselves. One day we all had cupcakes to eat in class, and people actually waited for me to wipe the table down before they started eating.

I was pretty sure my fellow students, as nice as they were, regarded me as a curiosity. But I didn't care. I was so happy to have human companionship after so long in isolation, I'd have wiped down the entire school if I'd had to.

As I was heading toward class one day, it started raining cats and dogs. Even for the Seattle region, this was an extraordinary amount of rain. As I made my way through the courtyard, I noticed an enormous puddle, and it brought me up short.

The thousands and thousands of raindrops hitting that puddle were creating ripples, and as the ripples fanned out, they made an interference pattern with the other ripples. I was transfixed by that beautiful example of the nature of things and found myself staring down as the ripples made their circular peaks and valleys and thousands of new raindrops erased them and made more. It reminded me of the inverse-square law of physics that I'd begun to learn about through my own research—in fact, it was a perfect example of the law that applies when some force or energy is radiated outward from a single point into three-dimensional space. As the energy gets farther from the source, it is spread across an area that is increasing proportionally to the source—and the energy is inversely proportional to the radius of the space. Though the concept was usually applied in the context of gravity, light, sound, radiation, or electricity, I saw the distribution pattern on the surface of the water as well.

I didn't have an umbrella, but I didn't care that I was dripping wet and that water was cascading off my head. It was not unpleasant at all. This was a late-summer day and the rain was lukewarm. I took a camera out of my suitcase and hunched over it to keep it dry. I stood photographing that remarkable display for some time, a huge grin on my face. I wanted to always remember it.

I don't know how much time had passed when I heard rapping on glass nearby. It was loud; I could hear it over the rain. When I looked up, I saw a group of students gathered behind the large glass wall ahead of me, laughing and talking and pointing at me. It looked like an entire class, including the professor, had interrupted their lesson in order to watch me.

It occurred to me how wet I was at that point and how strange I must look. One of the students snapped a picture, the flash briefly illuminating that gray afternoon. A bunch of students started waving at me. I waved back, and more pictures were taken. I smiled at them and laughed along with them, then continued on to my class.

When I got my photos developed, they weren't that great. They weren't as sharply focused or filled with wave patterns as the images I'd seen with my own eyes. Real life is so much better for me than photos; I think it's because motion creates additional effects in my perception that can't be captured by a camera. Flipping through a magazine one day on campus, I learned about some photography software called Genuine Fractals (now renamed Perfect Resize 7.5). This Photoshop plug-in allowed you to increase the resolution of a photo and reopen it in improved focus at almost any scale. I thought that sounded one step better than what I had, but I wished there were software that could capture precisely what I saw. Perhaps one day I could create it.

It didn't take my teachers long to discover I was no ordinary student. Though I was going to school only part-time so I could begin working again at Planet Futon, I was serious about my courses. I sat in the front of each classroom and raised my hand often. I noticed my professors looking at me oddly during my daily purification rituals and when I engaged them in class, and it was obvious that they found me not only unusual but perhaps exceptional — simultaneously deficient in mathematical terminology and fundamentals and extremely advanced in my theorizing. I made the effort to answer a lot of questions and ask new ones. There was a guy in one of my classes who clucked every time I did, but I wasn't going to let him get to me.

I started to be encouraged by the faculty members' inquisitiveness. They had questions for me, too, about how I thought and how I arrived at various answers. I got the feeling that despite my nontraditional methodology, I was coming up with the right answers and maybe even some surprising questions. I started sharing my drawings after class.

My introductory algebra teacher, Tracy Haynie, asked us to draw a nautilus from triangles based on a lesson in our textbook. The exercise required us to simply find the correct-size triangles to place in the outline of the shell in a flat, two-dimensional way, but I was inspired immediately when I saw it. I realized I could build a three-dimensional spiral nautilus like the one I'd loved in childhood if I applied the Pythagorean theorem. I drew the first triangle and then, using the equation $a^2 + b^2 = c^2$, I recursively put c back in the equation as a, kept b as one, and grew it out, kind of like how Mandelbrot formed his set. Placing each new triangle, calculated this way at a right angle to the first, grew out a perfect nautilus.

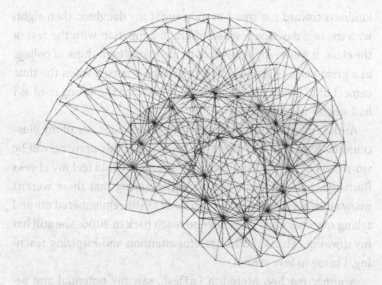

Haynie was fascinated enough to ask the other students to draw a seashell using the Pythagorean theorem, as I had. Mine was seventeen times larger than what she had them draw, but many of them were excited by the exercise and now we were all talking about it.

One day I was walking down the hall, struggling with my rolling suitcase and with my arms full of drawings. I was facing a troublesome hallway door that pulled inward (making my foot or elbow method unworkable). It also had a handicapped buzzer, but that was out of order. Haynie appeared out of nowhere, swooped in, and opened the door for me. I can't tell you what this simple act of kindness, followed by meaningful conversations about the OCD that kept me from touching door handles, meant to me coming from an instructor. She even said, "I think I have a little touch of that," and I believed her, since she kept her classroom so neat and tidy. Her reaction was so, well, human, it made me want to work even harder.

I felt very much at home and inspired by Haynie's class and her kindness toward me that I even brought my daughter, then eight, with me one day. She learned to graph a function with the rest of the class. It was really important to me that Megan think of college as a great place to go. I wanted her to apply herself when the time came. I didn't want her to lose time or go down the wrong road as I had when I was younger.

At the end of the semester, Haynie asked me for one of my illustrations. "One day you might be famous and this drawing will be worth lots of money," she said with a smile. I could feel my cheeks flush red. Later she sent me an e-mail saying that there weren't many students she remembered as well as she remembered me and telling me what a joy I had been to teach back in 2006. She still has my drawing. Thanks to her careful attention and inspiring teaching, I came to love school.

Another teacher, Meredith LaFlesh, saw my potential and zeroed in on me during her rotations in the math lab, tutoring me in trigonometry and filling in the blanks in my math vocabulary. I realized how fortunate I was to be connecting with great teachers and I tried to make the most of their generous attention. One night, freshly inspired by LaFlesh's instruction, I set out to create a formula describing pi and arrived at the following:

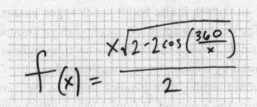

$$f(x) = \frac{x\sqrt{2 - 2\cos\left(\frac{360}{x}\right)}}{2}$$

I showed up early the next day and knocked on her door as soon as the light in her classroom flickered on. The legally blind LaFlesh put on her glasses—a pair with a very high degree of magnification — and studied my work. She typed the equation into her scientific calculator and brought it to within an inch of her eyes.

"This is correct!" she said, leaning back in her chair and looking at me with awe. "How did you do this?" I explained that I visualized pi as a shape in space and worked backward to find the formula that accurately represented it. I saw pi as a function of a circle subdivided by triangles where x equaled the number of triangles. As x approached infinity, $f(x)$ approached pi. She shook her head in wonder and had me work through each stage of the back-to-front calculation on the blackboard.

My reputation with the students began to improve as well. They were getting used to the fact that I was always raising my hand in class. A few of them told me I was asking the questions everyone else was too shy to ask. Even the nonstop partiers, who I suspected were always hung over in class, eventually warmed up to me, seeking me out at the math lab to ask me to explain the week's assignments with my drawings. I found myself counseling them, telling them I had been just like them when I was their age and that they ought to stay in more often and concentrate on their studies. I felt like I was talking to my younger self.

I loved the math lab. It was not only a place to go for supplemental help, but also a place where students could discuss and even debate important lessons. I tried to get past how grossed out I was by having to log in on a touchscreen computer — I wiped the glass off to do so and, later, the keyboard. Then there was the issue of the curious way questions were asked in the lab. There was a bowl in the front of each desk almost overflowing with marbles. Beside it was a silk daisy. You needed to pick up the daisy by the stem and stick it upright in the bowl to signal you needed help. I was so scared of this dust collector that I picked it up using one of my wipes every time. I tended to spill a bunch of marbles out of the bowl when I put the daisy in, as did my fellow students. Every time this happened, some people applauded. I usually felt so embarrassed for whoever had spilled the marbles — kind of the way I do when a waiter drops a glass in a restaurant. I never had such empathy before, but now it's literally a tightening in my chest. So the silence of that environment was punctuated by the spilling of marbles and huddled students discussing math.

I made some good friends there. One of my new admirers was so enthralled by my drawings he decided to show my illustration of pi to a tenured professor we ran into in the hallway. I hadn't yet been in any of this professor's classes, though I hoped to be soon, as he was one of the most respected teachers at the school. The professor looked it over and announced, "This is correct, but only someone who hasn't been taught how to think would calculate pi this way . . . who's the student? I have to meet him!"

"It's me," I said in a little mouse of a voice as I stood beside my friend. The professor smacked his hand to his head and bounced up and down a couple of times and said, "This is genius!" Then he shook my hand and asked me all about myself in the few minutes before the next class period. I walked away elated.

All the positive feedback I was getting in school made me realize that something really extraordinary was going on with me — that it was not just all in my head, so to speak. I started to hang around the student newspaper office to tell them about my unusual case. What I really wanted to do was share some of my drawings with the student community through the paper so I could teach more people about math from a visual point of view. The staff was very interested, and one reporter taped hours and hours of conversation. A story never appeared, however, and the newspaper ended up closing.

There were definitely some people at school who didn't understand me or get where I was coming from. There was the clucking fellow student in my trigonometry class, but he dropped out. He was quickly replaced in the math lab by a student who was very religious and looked at me warily whenever I described the world in geometric terms or by using the laws of physics. I don't disrespect people's beliefs, but he really had a problem with my secular approach. The instructors broke up our animated debates a couple of times.

There was also one instructor in the math lab who clearly was having a little fun with me. He called me the Math-Lab Janitor, because of the way I sanitized my workspace each day, and joked that the room had never been so clean. He would come by my desk over and over when I was working and put his finger on the Enter button of my scientific calculator just to watch me swab it down immediately with a baby wipe. I tried to smile through it and keep from telling him how truly terrified I was by those germs that he found so funny.

Perhaps the most difficult hurdle was the class on the use of calculus in physics. I was really excited to begin, as I felt this was where the lectures would get into the fine detail of why things are the way they are.

In the beginning, my biggest challenge was setting up the equations for the word problems; basically, changing a story into symbols. There were so many different variables and symbols that I didn't yet know, I worried that I'd never pass the class. When they were finally set up and it came down to doing the calculations, I was much more at ease.

It was a large class, and the instructor grumbled whenever I raised my hand to ask a question or make an observation. Although the majority of my teachers encouraged participation, there were a few sticklers who just wanted to make it through the syllabus without interruption or tangential inquiry.

One day we got into a discussion about instantaneous velocity, and I brought up that I had a problem with how calculus required the assumption that things approach infinity in order to get the result. I didn't think that was the correct way because that gave you only an approximation, in my humble opinion. I would much rather have calculated it this way:

True instantaneous velocity = change in position/Planck time.

I called the professor sir, and I tried to be polite, but he was clearly annoyed. He said something like "Grrr. Yes," granting my point but clearly wanting to move on. It was correct, and he acknowledged that, as bothered as he was by the interruption.

I continued to remain engaged in my classes despite these hurdles. However, one teacher dealt me a near-fatal academic blow.

A new professor was working in the math lab. While discussing a math problem with him, I explained that I needed to visualize it as shapes first before I went to the next step. He looked at me with a really perplexed face and said, "Well, there's something wrong with your brain, then."

I felt a dagger go deep into my heart. My ears started to get warm with shame and I tried to explain how ever since my injury, I'd automatically associated shapes with numbers. Now they were encoded in my mind, I continued, and helped me with memory and calculations. Have you ever heard of synesthesia? I asked him.

"You need a new brain. Numbers are *not* shapes," he retorted.

I was silenced. I was so shocked and ashamed that I wished I could run and hide behind the blanketed windows of my home. But then shame gave way to anger. I gathered my books and drawings and went to the head of the math department. The man was one of my calculus teachers, the best of the bunch, and he listened intently as I described the insulting conversation I'd just had.

"He belittled me," I said. "He wouldn't even listen to me so I could show him my system would still yield the right answer."

He had sympathy for me and said he was wrong and that it shouldn't have happened. "But before you file a report, I need to tell you something," he said. "He just found out he has cancer."

I was stunned. I felt so sorry for him. I thought of the loss of my own beloved stepfather to the disease and immediately changed my mind about filing a report.

His words still stung me, though, and I realized that although math abilities came easily to me now, the path ahead of me in legitimizing these abilities and getting a formal education was going to be a challenging one. The euphoria I felt in returning to school was tempered with caution now and perhaps that was for the best. I resolved to continue to work as hard as I could, unaware I'd have a new reason to be joyful in the coming weeks.

CHAPTER TEN

The Hermit and the Hermitage

LUNCH TRAYS WERE clanging, people were speaking to my left and my right, and announcements were coming over the public-address system, but I didn't hear a thing. I was sitting at the cafeteria table at Tacoma Community College and drawing intensely, deeply absorbed in getting every line perfect. I was in the zone and had noticed that when I needed to work, I was able to project the safe, quiet space I'd created for myself during my years of isolation around me like a protective bubble. I was surprised, as I'd never had this ability before, and in the old days, I would have been holding court at one of the tables, describing last night's debauchery or planning that night's.

I barely noticed when a young woman sat at the last seat available, two places to my right. From bits of conversation I heard over the din, I became vaguely aware that she knew the other young woman directly to my right and that they had a German class together. I finished my drawing, checked my watch, and saw that I had a few minutes left before class. I decided to talk to the woman nearest me. I began to show her my drawings, but it was her friend who told me she thought they were amazing; she said that her father was an engineer and had drafted similar patterns and blueprints while she was growing up. She asked me how I managed to draw them. I told her I used a ruler and sometimes a compass.

"My dad had tools like that too!" she said excitedly, then looked down, a shy person catching herself in a moment of enthusiasm.

I stared at her a little longer than I ordinarily would have, since her eyes were averted, and I immediately wanted to know more about him and more about her as well. I felt an unfamiliar but instant intimacy at her comparing my work to her dad's.

I asked her where she was from — her accent was charming.

"I'm from Russia."

"I'm from Alaska!" I responded, feeling a strong connection that I wasn't sure was just about the neighboring geography.

"Do you know Alaska used to be part of Russia?" she asked.

"Yes, I do."

Her name was Elena Afanasyeva and she was a dual major, business and finance. Elena looked like a snow maiden, with porcelain skin and pale blond hair cut in a bob. Her eyes were lit with intelligence, and her voice was gentle and soft. She seemed genuinely interested in my work. I tried not to stare at her. I realized I'd been alone too long.

I may have been a very confident guy in my glory days but it had been years since any woman had responded to me like that. In the past, I was now aware, my interactions with women were largely based on physical attraction, aided by some clever conversation that certainly didn't rise to the level of the things that occupied my mind now.

I was not that man anymore — the one to whom relationships, albeit mostly superficial ones, came so easily — and I was adrift. I felt shy and I worried that Elena would see right through me and know the wreck I'd been since the mugging. With my physical difficulties — my neck and back were still affected by the beating I took — I had not worked out in years. I knew I was getting ahead of myself, but I could see that she was fascinated by my drawings, and I allowed myself to think for a second that if she was that interested in the only thing I really cared about now, we might actually have a chance to be more than friends. In fact, I was glad I was currently single and alone. The loneliness had been hard to bear, but it meant I was available. It was as though fate had put me in a holding pattern for just this moment.

Snapping out of my reverie, I realized it was almost time for me to get to my next class. I knew I wanted to see her again but I couldn't bring myself to ask her out in the few minutes I had left, and I brooded over my atrophied social skills all the way down the hall. Right as I was about to kick open the door to the classroom, something told me to turn around, and I ran back to the courtyard and gave Elena my number on a small slip of paper. She looked at me like, *Are you kidding me?* I left feeling dejected, and then three days later, the phone rang.

Megan handed me the receiver and it was Elena; she wanted to know if I would like to go to a soccer game that some of her South American friends, also international students at our school, were putting together in a few hours. Wow, would I *ever*, I thought. But with my daughter standing right in front of me, I felt I had to explain who'd picked up the phone and tell Elena a little more about myself first. "Can my daughter come? She's with me today. I think she'd enjoy watching the game."

"Of course" came the faint reply.

I needed to know from the start that Elena would be okay with my daughter. I didn't know until she told me later that it was a shock at first and that she worried I had too much history for her to deal with.

I'd thought for years that I would never resume a normal social life and it was hard to let go of that fear, but something in Elena's voice on the phone was so comforting and warm that it was easy for me to segue from asking her how school was going to discussing other light topics. Though I felt guilty about it, I decided not to take Megan to the game. If things went well, Elena would meet Megan eventually. For that day, I wanted to be able to focus all my attention on Elena. I arranged for Megan's favorite sitter and went on to meet Elena at a bus stop near the school. She was joined by her best friend, a Chilean student named Carolina. As the soccer game commenced, I found myself sharing all I could with Elena in the stands — about what happened the night of the mugging, about my drawings, about the geometry I saw all around me. I was afraid I might be overwhelming her, but I thought it was important that she knew who I was from the start. To my delight, she smiled and nodded a lot and asked plenty of her own questions about my theories. Bonus: she was really bright and had a quirky, sharp sense of humor that was some blend of American and Russian sensibility I found really intriguing.

Our conversation continued through the game and over pizza afterward. I couldn't believe how connected I felt to this woman. I am ashamed to say it, but when she told me she was twenty, I fibbed and told her I was twenty-eight instead of the truth, that I was thirty-five. I was already afraid of losing her.

We started doing more things together. Soon, it was as interesting for me to be out of the house as in it. I was just as obsessed with math and science as before, but now I didn't have to sit alone with it; I had someone to discuss it with who really cared. We went to a party at her friend Carolina's house and I guided her through the crowd, making very detailed observations about the body language of various people as they appeared to me, something I realized might be a new obsession since I was back in public. But she didn't find it strange. On each date, I showed her a few more of my tics, waiting for her to run for the hills. Instead, she accepted me and began to share more about herself. But we'd yet to be totally alone.

I asked her to a movie and she said yes. About two-thirds of the way through it I took her hand and held it. I had butterflies. I tried to kiss her that night but she turned her head. It was okay — for this special woman, I'd be willing to wait as long as I had to.

For our next date, we took Megan to Seattle for the day. The two of them got along really well. This was so important to me and a big step forward. I washed my convertible and asked Elena before we set off if she minded having the top down. I wanted to make sure she'd be comfortable with the wind blowing her hair around. She was game, and about halfway through the trip, as we cruised down the highway, she threw her head back and told me that it felt like heaven.

I knew I wanted to invite her to our home at that point, so I set a date two weeks out. I'd have liked it to be sooner, but I thought about my place, with the papers and drawings piled high every-where, and I knew it was going to take a while to clean. It was not like there were moldy plates of food lying around — it was germ-free, given my cleanliness phobia — but it looked like a birdcage freshly lined with drawings of pi. And, oh, the hole in the roof with the pigeons flying in and out. I was nearly red with embarrassment even though she couldn't see the picture I was conjuring in my mind. I'd have to call my cousin to do a low-cost but total rehab on the place before Elena came over.

We spent the next two weeks getting the place Elena-worthy. My cousin and I repaired the hole in the roof, the siding, and the wonky doorbell, working seven days a week. I organized my papers, sepa-rating my own work from Megan's school projects. I was a hoarder when it came to my daughter's creations and I kept every one of them.

The day of Elena's visit arrived. I cut the lawn and washed my car and then went to a Russian florist I'd found to see about getting the right flowers. I was surprised to learn that in Elena's culture, *even* numbers of flowers are presented only for sympathy or funeral arrangements. I still bought a dozen red roses, but I put eleven in a vase and handed her one when she came to the door. I had ordered take-out and had a rented movie ready. She looked nervous at first, but then we got to talking, and our chemistry was easy and obvious. Over dinner, Elena said she understood how hard it had been for me. She said she liked both the person I'd been and the person I'd become. For my part, I realized that my old self never would have been good enough for Elena, and my paradoxical feelings about the outcome of the mugging now also included an unexpected infusion of gratitude.

It wasn't until Elena started spending more time with me that I realized how much I had been missing in recent years. I had been without much human companionship or happiness. While she was a serious student and every bit my intellectual equal, Elena had no interest in sitting at home and just thinking, going up and down scientific rabbit holes. She inspired me to look outside of my own mind for destinations, to engage with my surroundings and achieve a balance between exploring my new abilities and finding their place in the wider world.

I wanted to return the favor. Elena hadn't seen much of the United States yet. She'd been busy getting straight A's at our college, which she'd chosen because it had a good program for international students and she wanted to learn more English. She grew up enamored of the American soap *Santa Barbara*. The influence of that show in Russia was like *Dallas*'s in its heyday here in the States, and for Elena, it defined American culture. She had planned to travel to the actual Southern California city with Carolina, but her best friend had returned to Chile. I decided to step in and start making some of her dreams come true if at all possible. Getting her to Santa Barbara was easy. "I'll take you," I said, and she threw her arms around me. I couldn't believe how good that felt. When Elena's face lit up, I felt like I could fly. It helped to have someone to focus on besides me. It felt good to make someone else happy.

We made plans to see some of the iconic sights of the city and bought tickets to Disneyland as well. But when we arrived, Elena came down with the worst stomach pains she'd ever had. We didn't know if it was one too many fast-food hamburgers or the sheer excitement of the journey, but she was down for the count. I realized how much I'd grown to love her as I nursed her in our hotel room and honestly didn't give a second thought to the vacation plans. My only concern was for Elena, who recovered in time to catch a few highlights of the planned journey.

As we began our abbreviated tour of Santa Barbara, we stopped at a light at one of the main intersections. Just as a slightly queasy Elena was starting to ooh and aah at the places she recognized from her favorite series, a fight broke out between two motorists behind us in traffic. So much for the idealized American mythology of the TV show, I thought. Elena and I flagged down a nearby police officer, who quickly jumped into the melee and arrested the guys. We pulled away laughing at the unfortunate interruption of the fantasy.

Our time in Santa Barbara was largely spent tooling around in the car with Elena jumping out to take photos at the locations she recognized. When she began to tire, we called it a day. She needed to rest for Disneyland.

We made our way to the Anaheim amusement park, and Elena confessed she'd never been on a roller coaster before. That had to be remedied, queasy stomach or not, I told her. She was a real sport and decided to join me for the enormous California Screamin' coaster. She squeezed my hand really tight as they locked us in, and we began our ride.

At that point, I realized I had not been on a roller coaster since the brain injury. It was too late to back out and I was really apprehensive. As the cart sped through the loops and up the humongous inclines and back down them with increasing velocity, the stop-action frames I was used to seeing for motion flew by at an amazing clip. I couldn't believe how exciting this was. I whooped and hollered at every twist and turn. Elena closed her eyes for the worst of it but was beaming when we exited, having checked *ride roller coaster* off her list of American things to do.

Not long after the trip I decided to tell her the truth about my age. I explained that I'd thought we'd never have a chance if I told her the truth at the outset, before we got to know each other. She stared at me stone-faced and said, "Drive me home."

For the next three days in school she wouldn't even look at me. I was distraught. But on the third day, she pulled me aside and took my hand. She'd been thinking about it and she realized she loved me despite the age difference and the deception. Holding back tears, I promised never to lie to her again. I told her I loved her too. For the first time in my life, I was in a serious relationship and I wasn't afraid of where things were headed. I knew we belonged together.

The semester ended all too soon and Elena had to return home to Russia. Before leaving, she admitted she'd known it was serious that first day at the soccer match. In the beginning, she explained, she thought she was going to be in America for only a few months of studying and she figured she should take the opportunity to get to know as many interesting people as possible. But apparently, she had strong feelings for me. "I felt safe," she told me. "And I always love people who have a passion in their life, as you clearly did. I could tell you were fascinated by these important ideas and it made me see the world differently. I'd never met anyone like you."

I drove her to the airport. Our farewell was so full of tears that people around us in the terminal looked upset. We were both sobbing and clinging to each other, not wanting to let go. Elena said it first — there was no way of telling if the geography would be a permanent barrier. And if it caused long separations between us, who was to say we wouldn't both meet other people?

The instant she disappeared behind the gate, I knew I would go to Russia to win her hand. There would be no stopping me. Reality solidified, and all the different potentials for my life became one point. On the drive home, I actually felt my spirits lift because of this certainty about what I must do. And in the following very long days without her, I began making arrangements for my first overseas journey. I'd go to Russia and convince her to live in the States permanently.

Still, when I really thought about it, making the trip seemed impossible. It hadn't been that long ago that I'd been hiding behind my windows with blankets over them, completely isolated. Getting on that plane to a strange place so far away would be one of the hardest things I'd ever do. But my feelings for Elena trumped everything else, and I did it.

We arranged for her to travel from her small town of Pskov to St. Petersburg to pick me up at the airport. This was a four-hour journey over rough terrain by bus, not to mention the long walk to the bus station she had to make from her town to begin the trip. I was worried for her and worried we'd miss each other.

The plane landed, and I picked up my luggage and then went to the customs agent to get checked through. Something was apparently wrong with the way I'd filled out my customs declaration, however, and pretty soon there were three agents, all speaking to me mostly in Russian. I had no idea what was going on. I saw passenger after passenger being let through; an hour later, I was still there with the customs agents. I worried that by now Elena would think I stood her up and she'd leave. Down the hall from me was a window. I was not sure if Elena would be on the other side of it but I bolted to it and waved.

Elena was feeling dejected as she asked the last straggling passengers if there was anyone left behind them. They said no and then expressed sympathy. Miraculously, she saw me waving and asked to be let in to help me. The guards who followed me down the hall when I ran were only too anxious to speak with her by this time. She cleared up the mistakes I'd made on the form and we were let go; we left and headed to the hotel where we planned to spend a couple of nights before continuing on to her town.

When we exited the airport and made our way to the city, I found myself overwhelmed by all the new shapes of the architecture and the other sights and sounds and even the unfamiliar aromas. From the gilded cupola of St. Isaac's Cathedral to the domes, spires, and intricate mosaics of the Church of Our Savior on Spilled Blood, traditional Russian architecture was so ornate that I could hardly take my eyes off the extra geometrical angles. Even the modern, huge, and boxy apartment complexes were on such a large scale that I found myself staring at the seemingly endless numbers of windows on their facades. I was used to seeing my own complicated geometrical imagery, but to have real, solid, complex, and new forms to consider was very discomfiting.

As happy as I was to be reunited with Elena, the smog created by the old cars of the fallen empire burned my eyes and stung my throat. And there was rust everywhere; time and again, I was offended by its presence on things that must have once been so beautiful. I retreated to the hotel room at one point and went to my safe space, staring at the water coming out of the faucet in the bathroom sink like I did every morning at home. I thought if I kept my normal routines I wouldn't be so addled, but when I looked at my webby water forms for some sort of comfort, I realized the water was yellow and smelled of sulfur. There was no use hiding in the boxy room either, as room service delivered one strange dish after another, and nothing on TV made sense. I noticed that alphabet graphics in the news reports were different from English and quickly turned the television off, stung by the letters' shapes.

Worse than that, my eyes began to hurt, and my whole body bristled at the new landscapes. It was a feeling of being closed in; I felt like the buildings were leaning in toward me and I was trapped in a canyon. It took me a few days to adjust to the new forms; this odd, new structure of things was overwhelming. It was as if I could feel my brain growing new neurons to adapt to my surroundings. I realized I was acquiring a totally new definition of what a city looked like. As stimulating as these images were, it was still the overlay of shapes I saw synesthetically and my acquired savant response to them that left me the most fascinated and started to make me feel at home.

I remember seeing a train go by in St. Petersburg. There was a man leaning out the window of one of the cars, smoking. When the choppy frames of the train going by and the new landscape behind it became overwhelming for me, I focused instead on the puffs of smoke around the man. The little particles I saw within the swirls of smoke were also swirling or darting within the cloud. I'd seen this before, even while avoiding smokers on sidewalks back home, and just that tiny detail grounded me again.

I would find even greater comfort looking at the Velikaya River in Pskov. Standing on a bridge above it one day, I saw the waves of the water interfering with one another as they flowed past the cement support columns below me. It reminded me of the physics double-slit experiment, in which photons can interfere with one another while acting as waves. To me, it was reminiscent of a drawing I had done, and the very memory of the illustration comforted me greatly in this new environment.

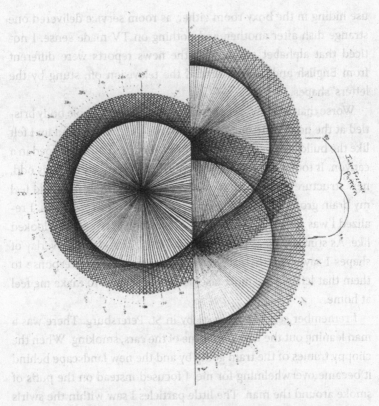

I tried to escape to these familiar visions when I was uncomfortable. Even if something was very beautiful, I found it could overwhelm me. This was never more clear than when Elena took me to the Hermitage, the former Winter Palace of the czars that's now a treasure-filled art museum. She later said our time there was classic Jason. I suppose it was.

We were walking in a gallery filled with eighteenth-century portraits. The ceilings soared and the archways were enormous. It was gilded — no expense had been spared in its creation. The paintings were also oversize; anything smaller than those gigantic canvases would have been utterly lost in that space. Elena was feeling great pride in her heritage and carefully paused at each face or faces, explaining to me the history behind them. We were so important to each other by then that I knew she wanted me to not just see the paintings but feel them, to know her through them. However, I was distracted, and I kept looking over my shoulder. She told me later how it hurt to lose my attention. She tried to emphasize certain points louder and look in my eyes directly to hold my gaze, but it was no use. I couldn't help it. I walked away, down the hallway, where I ended up with my face about an inch away from a mirror hanging there. I'm not usually that rude. Elena followed me down the hall and asked what I was doing.

"Elena," I said, all seriousness. "Do you see the way the light is reflecting off this mirror? It's so beautiful." Though I had seen and even been obsessed with light playing off glass and mirrors before, the scale of the mirror as well as the enormous window letting the light in created the most elaborate, incredible, prismatic fanning-out of light rays I'd ever seen.

I learned later this light play is known in Italian as *gibigianna*, which translated to "charming woman." It certainly charmed me.

It was not that I didn't appreciate the collections in the Hermitage. But something in me saw more beauty, more value, in the natural and geometric underpinnings of the world. I may have had treasures untold at my feet in that moment, but they paled by comparison.

We made our way to Pskov and I gained even more appreciation and affection for Elena when I realized the difficulty of the journey she made to meet me. Compared to St. Petersburg, Pskov was pristine and reminded me of some of the small towns I'd lived in in Alaska. I'd arranged to rent a small flat about a mile from Elena's apartment. Her parents' place was too small for another person and they didn't know me yet. I vowed to win her parents over.

Elena's mom and dad were very kind to me from the start, and Elena translated patiently as we got to know one another. Through them, I saw the fall of the empire. Her father had lost his government engineering job in the breakup of the Soviet Union. He spoke briefly of having worked at Chernobyl after the nuclear meltdown and how he hadn't felt well since then. But he mostly talked about what happened to one of his friends. The colleague found a wristwatch in the largely abandoned town of Chernobyl and carried it around in his pants pocket for a couple of days. One day when he stripped to bathe, he noticed the skin on his leg under the watch had turned completely black.

Later, Elena told me that during Joseph Stalin's purges, her father's family home was burned. I felt nothing but sympathy for these people I'd been raised to fear during the Cold War. (Her father has since passed away.)

Elena's mother somehow managed to be the most lively, pleasant woman I'd ever met despite the great hardships she'd faced raising a child during the fall of an empire. Despite her formidable, serious beginnings — she was one of the few female software engineers of her generation, and she had had to be tough to achieve that position — she was always lighthearted and cheerful. She told me that when she'd started in the industry, a single computer took up an entire room. She had seen so much. It didn't matter if she was on a breadline or working as an engineer in a power plant that had no heat and, at one point, no roof overhead. She met each challenge with great personal strength and sacrificed a lot for Elena, particularly after Elena's father grew ill. She reminded me of a little brown bird I'd once seen in Alaska. I was stacking supplies on a huge metal shelf in an industrial yard near the oil fields when I disturbed a nest filled with eggs. The mother bird swooped, then flopped to the ground and pretended to have a broken wing to pull my attention to her. I'd walk toward the mother bird, away from the eggs, and she'd fly back to the nest, and then she'd repeat the swooping and flopping when I approached the shelving and the nest again. Like that bird, Elena's mom would risk anything to give her daughter a chance, would even work in unsafe conditions to support her family. Most remarkably, she never passed on any inner fear she might have had to her child. (She recently retired, after thirty-six years with the same employer.)

Meeting Elena and her family changed my worldview. The geometry of the relationships among and within nations would never be the same for me. The lines that were borders on world maps faded in my mind.

Despite the bleak surroundings and stories, I'd gone to Russia to win Elena, and so I decided I would bring as much joy as possible into her life while I was there. One of the first things I did was take Elena and two of her girlfriends bowling. This may be considered a blue-collar activity in the States, but it's a really posh thing to do in the former Soviet Union, and I wanted to impress her. Things were going well until a drunk Russian police officer approached our group and said something about the women.

Elena translated for me and I could smell the vodka on his breath as he teetered and glared. All I could think of was ending up in the gulag. According to Elena, he was challenging me to a bowling match. *At least it's not pistols at ten paces,* I thought.

I had seen a large, framed portrait of the reigning champion of the lane on my way in. The smiling man was surrounded by a CD player and other loot he'd won in their biggest competition. It said his average was a 160. Mine was a 200 back when I bowled. I quickly calculated that if the cop was a regular here and had been beaten by this guy, I had a chance.

"Tell him I'll bowl against him, Elena," I said.

With that, the cop's eyes lit up and he reached for a bowling ball. He raised it over his head and began whipping it around in a circular fashion, shouting things that were lost to our translation system because we ducked instead of talking.

Just as the ball was on the downward curve behind his head, momentum and gravity took over, and the policeman fell flat on his back. We tried not to laugh but it was the funniest thing I'd ever seen. I kept my head down so no one could see my big grin.

A second policeman approached our group, warned me not to kick his friend when he was down, and dragged him out of sight. Our date resumed.

Part of the fun of traveling to Russia was meeting the people and learning to appreciate their challenges. I realized that there were vast differences between the middle and upper classes when I had to stand on a long, snaking line just to buy a bottle of water one day (members of the upper class never had to wait in lines). Just when I got to the front of the line, the cashier closed the register down and pulled a chain across it. Elena told me I should have stepped to the front of a second line that had formed, just jam myself in there like everyone else, but it didn't feel polite to me.

I got to meet a man named Vladimir, a neighbor of Elena's family, who'd made a lot of money under mysterious circumstances in the new Russia and who enjoyed the power and privilege that goes with wealth. Our encounter happened just as it was nearly time for me to return to the States. Elena and I were standing outside my flat waiting for a taxi she'd called, as I would be staying in her family's apartment for my last night.

We'd handed the keys over to my landlady, and we had to stand in the thirty-below weather in our parkas for a few moments until the cab arrived. When the driver got a look at the big red satchel I was carrying he said, "Too big," and sped off.

We ended up having to walk in the frigid cold until we stumbled upon another cab by the side of the road. We arrived at her parents' apartment building with ice crystals on our eyelashes.

Stepping out of the shadows near the entrance to the building was the largest man I had ever seen.

"Lena, what has happened? Why do you two look so cold?" he

asked her in his booming baritone. She explained our harrowing tale and how we could have died out in the subzero weather.

"Give me the name of the cab company," said the man, who I would later learn was Vladimir. "I will handle this."

We learned the next day that not only had Vladimir gotten the driver fired, but the company withheld his Christmas bonus as well. The hulking Russian took a real shine to me on subsequent visits and bear-hugged me, slapped me on the back, and said, "I served in Cuba with the Soviet army, Jason! We are neighbors!"

I would end up making four journeys to Russia before I convinced Elena she should return with me to the States and be my wife.

I would have liked my proposal to have been more romantic, but it actually took place over the phone during one of our reluctant separations between visits. I told her I couldn't bear to be apart from her and wanted to build a future with her in America.

We were married on January 16, 2009, in Tacoma's city hall with no one but a Planet Futon employee and the employee's mother for witnesses. We were so happy — and so nervous — that we forgot to put batteries in our camera and have no photographs of the day.

In the trajectory of our love affair, I learned to trust and open up to the world again. Elena saved me in every sense of the word. I finally had someone to live the unmathematical angles of my life with and share my deepest hopes. And so there were two new things I loved now: geometry and my Elena. I returned to work with greater purpose, wanting to build a better life with her.

CHAPTER ELEVEN

The Man from Planet Futon

I WAS TRANSFORMED NOW that I had Elena to share my life. I couldn't believe my good fortune most days as we planned our future, including starting our own family. With her encouragement, I was a little more relaxed around people and out in public. It had been seven years since the attack. It was still not easy at the store sometimes, because you never really knew who would walk in.

It was funny to remember, given my skittishness about dealing with the public, that when I started selling futons out of my home in Alaska in the early 1990s, I had let all types of people through the front door for the sake of a sale. It was a far cry from the flagship Planet Futon store we would open in Tacoma in 2001. Back then, I ran a Yellow Pages ad and let customers come over at all hours to see the two models of futons from my dad's factory I had set up in my living room. I was partying a lot in those days, but despite all the time I spent away from home or recovering from long nights out, I had a good business going. I was able to pay my rent and all my bills and put a good sum aside. It wasn't long before I had enough saved to rent a little store in the local Anchorage mall big enough to display ten futons. I named that store Futon Gallery. Those were the golden days of futons. The popular TV show *Friends* caused a run on the item because there was one on its set. The things practically sold themselves, sort of like waterbeds did back in the day.

I used to show up at the mall late — or whenever I wanted, really. The malls didn't fine you the way they do today if you don't open on time. I enjoyed the customers, especially the women. I would pretend not to know which futon they were referring to just so I could whip out a muscular arm and point at pieces of the inventory. I can't tell you how many times a pretty young woman would say, "Oh, look at your muscles. Can I touch them?" And of course I'd let her, because that was the point in the first place.

But since the brain injury, I could not stand anyone except Elena and Megan touching me. As soon as a customer came in the store, I started sizing up his hygiene and homing in on where he put his hands, what he touched, if he touched the people he came in with, where he touched them, and which hand he covered his mouth with if he coughed or sneezed. I tried to keep at least two feet of space between a customer and me at all times and if anyone came an inch closer, I backed up.

I knew that I looked uneasy so I tried to explain to some of them that I had profound OCD as a result of an accident. Most of them nodded but I don't think many of them understood.

In addition to being hyperaware of customers' germs, I would not turn my back on any of them, out of fear they would try to hurt me. This was part of the posttraumatic stress disorder from the mugging, no doubt. As I was scanning customers for evidence of germs, I was also looking for signs of potential violence. Many victims of traumatic brain injury suffer from an inability to understand nonverbal communication, such as body language. I was obsessed with interpreting people's behavior, so this wasn't a problem for me.

I'd had a couple of Skype conversations with the savant syndrome expert Dr. Treffert by now. It meant the world to me that the man I'd seen on television in the report about autistic savant and synesthete Daniel Tammet, which helped me know I was not completely alone, had become a guide as I navigated these waters. I hoped to meet him in person one day, but it would require taking time off from the store and flying to Fond du Lac, Wisconsin. Dr. Treffert is so revered in the field that people fly from all over the world — even the Far East — to his beautiful little midwestern town to see him. He explained that my intense focus on body language could be attributed to the increase in sensitivity and awareness that many acquired savants experience. He asked me a lot of questions because he was worried my sensitivity to other people's behaviors might be compulsive. After discussing it with me, he said, "Sometimes the increased sensitivity is a gift and sometimes a burden, again, depending on how intrusive it becomes. In your case I would list this as a plus, and not a tradeoff."

It *was* mostly a plus, but sometimes it was a burden too. I began to notice that when I was with people, if someone was uncomfortable, I was often aware of that person's discomfort long before anyone else in the room noticed. Or I'd sense someone's boredom with whatever subject was being talked about. When I felt someone else's embarrassment or boredom, I tried to change the subject or somehow change the dynamic of what was going on. Just like having OCD, it was a lot of work and a lot of worrying and very tiring to be on guard for not only myself but everyone around me at all times. I think Dr. Treffert would categorize that part as obsessive. So it did sometimes go into the negative area. If I had to rank the hierarchy of conditions in my head, I'd say that empathy trumped my aversion to germs in most cases — I didn't want to make other people uncomfortable by obviously avoiding touching them. But sometimes my OCD did battle with my empathy when I applied antibacterial lotion on my skin right after shaking hands with someone. I knew I might embarrass people but I just couldn't help it, and I would apologize profusely. When I thought about it, I realized I'd begun saying "I'm sorry" an awful lot.

I was still having difficulty with written forms of communication. (Except when it had to do with math research; the obsessive drive to know more about math, particularly geometry, got me over any inability or lack of desire to read or write.) It was very frustrating to me because it was such a crucial part of my schooling and I needed the skills for business. But at the same time, I had this heightened sensitivity to nonverbal cues. Why wasn't my whole ability to communicate wiped out? According to Greg Ayotte, the director of consumer services for the Brain Injury Association of America, communication is no longer believed to be localized in a particular part of the brain, and diffuse areas may get rewired and take over. State-of-the-art brain scans have shown that this sort of rewiring can happen in TBI survivors.

The hyperaware parts of me were a new positive for my work at my current store, Planet Futon, in the sense that I could plan my sales approach from the moment customers arrived. I'd had plenty of practice with salesmanship since we'd opened the store in 2001, but since my brain injury, I found myself better able to read people. For example, if a sedan pulled up — no sale. A minivan was more likely to be a serious customer, and a pickup truck was a sure bet. If a couple walked in, I'd focus on the less open of the two, monitoring cues like crossed arms, which signaled being closed off. If they had kids and were buying bunk beds, I'd try to get them to upgrade to better memory-foam mattresses, knowing most parents will do anything for their children.

Tacoma is not as economically prosperous as Seattle. There are a lot of people struggling to get by. I tried to meet them halfway by offering a no-credit-check policy. I made an arrangement with a finance company that would help customers with their purchases if they could provide proof of employment and had checking accounts.

This began to draw in some hard-luck types who couldn't make purchases at the bigger stores, and while I was really happy to be helping people, we took our share of hits from being so open. One woman bounced a check she wrote to us and when I phoned her, she said, "That's impossible, I still have two checks left on the account!" Another woman was about to bounce her check and the bank called me; I deposited the forty-dollar difference so our sale would go through. The customer phoned me furious that her account had been wiped out, though she'd received a forty-dollar discount. When I explained that intentionally taking merchandise and writing a bad check on it was just like stealing, she said, "Oh, you big companies can afford it."

I had enjoyed sales much more in the past. So much of my time was now taken up policing things. But that didn't mean it never got interesting. My best moments in the store became those spent talking about math and science, even with people who weren't going to buy anything. It was a real joy to see people's faces light up when they understood something, and I'd have to hone my own expertise on things when they asked difficult questions. Oftentimes I'd spend the rest of the evening reading things related to our conversations. It was one of my greatest pleasures to learn something new this way. It occurred to me that if I didn't have an outlet to discuss this with the general public, I'd probably go mad. I purposely turned conversations to the subjects that interested me just to get through the day.

I was alone in the furniture store one day when a brick wall of an ex-con walked in with his girlfriend and her two kids. "I want to know what's so good about this store. They say you have deals. I need a bed," the towering, totally bald man said. Though slight of build now, I thought back to my own days as a gym rat and figured the man weighed somewhere around 260 pounds, most of it muscle. I noticed the prison tattoos running up and down his arms.

"I'm Jason, and I can help you," I said nervously, still on guard with strangers.

"I'm Jason too," the customer replied. We chuckled at the coincidence, and the ice was broken. I couldn't help myself after that. I launched into my life story and apologized for being distracted when he first walked in. I told the man that ever since being mugged, I preferred to think about math and science over just about anything else, futons included. The brain injury I suffered appeared to have given me unexpected gifts, I offered.

The customer was staring wide-eyed. "I strong-arm-robbed a lot of people, but I never made nobody smarter!" He admitted he needed the bed because he'd just gotten out of prison and didn't have one waiting for him at home. I caught myself swallowing hard and slow. "You know the worst part about being in prison?" the parolee asked. I shook my head.

"I didn't get to smile for a year. I had to look mean. And I love to smile, don't I?" He looked toward his girlfriend while her kids jumped up and down on a nearby mattress. She laughed.

I started showing the man bed frames and box springs, walking backward to keep him in my line of sight. Trying not to stumble or look scared, I directed the conversation back to one of my comfort zones: the mathematical concept of pi. "Do you know that circles don't actually exist? If you zoom in close enough, their perimeters are actually zigzags — hundreds and hundreds of tiny little straight lines that are so close together they visually blend into a smooth curve from our perspective."

"For real?" Big Jason asked.

I went further, describing how if you fill in a circle with triangles, you can better measure its area, because there really is no curve to it at all. As I continued with the impromptu lecture, my customer's eyes lit up with understanding. I was thrilled to see that look on his face.

I carried on with the Doppler effect: "Imagine you're on one street corner and I'm on the next, and a car is speeding past both of us," I said. "I'll hear it as one pitch and you'll hear it as another, and overall it'll make that weird *nyeeeeeeruh* sound."

The customer nodded. "I've heard that sound."

"The pitch is relative to your position in space."

"That's all it is?" Big Jason looked scandalized. Then he reached into his pockets. "Don't you hate it when you spend time with a customer and they don't buy nothing?" the giant man teased.

"N-n-no, it's okay," I stammered. I was thinking I didn't care if the man bought anything as long as he left the store without hurting me. The customer pulled out a handful of wadded-up hundred-dollar bills and threw them on the mattress in front of us. "Well, I got the cash," he said with a smile. I sold him a king-size mattress and frame for a thousand dollars.

The man shook my hand and it was all I could do not to turn around and use the economy-size bottle of hand sanitizer behind the counter.

"I come to Planet Futon for a bed and I get life lessons," the ex-con said, his girlfriend and her kids trailing him out the door. "No circles, *wow* . . ."

I quickly washed my hands, then locked the store, hurried out the back, and ran down the street to deposit the money in the bank, looking over my shoulder every thirty seconds. Big Jason hadn't followed me.

I slowed my pace and as I walked toward the parking lot, I glanced up at the sunset and noticed the curvature of the sky. The half-dome shape began to divide itself into triangles, the figures sliding into place and glowing in the twilight. The streetlamps flickered on, and their light rays fanned out into perfect circles before filling up with the same procession of subdividing triangles. I watched the traffic go by in a slipstream, the images trailing one another like a stack of Polaroids.

My heart was still beating fast. I almost never felt completely out of danger interacting with that somewhat threatening stranger, but at least I completed the sale. That was a big moment for me and a sign of how far I'd come since my reclusive days.

Another day, I was delighted when a very clean, well-dressed man of about fifty entered the store. He looked a lot more promising than most of my customers and I felt that he was neither unhygienic nor dangerous. It turned out he was a pastor.

This gave me pause. My only association with organized religion until then was the Baptist church I'd attended with my grandparents for a time in Anchorage. They were evangelicals and there was a lot of threatening fire and brimstone shouted from that church pulpit that scared me away from their vengeful deity. Furthermore, the church battled the community where our home was, Hillside, by placing an illegal antenna in our neighborhood for their radio broadcasts. My mom headed the community group fighting to get it removed and was ultimately successful. Congregants started showing up in our front yard, cutting down tree branches and carting away our decorative stones for revenge. I was not a total disbeliever and knew not every congregation was like that; however, this had all soured me on being a churchgoer.

The pastor was a polite and friendly man. I guess cleanliness really is next to godliness, as the saying goes, because he looked so fresh and pure, even by my exacting standards. I found myself sharing my story and listening patiently as he talked about the miraculous nature of my recovery. I told him I couldn't argue that it was truly remarkable I was still walking around, much less experiencing my extraordinary new perspective, but I also told him that I had my share of questions about divinity being behind this. "I mean, if there is a God, didn't the same deity who might be responsible for my amazing new life also allow me to be beaten to within an inch of my life in the first place?" I asked.

"I have questions too," the graying visitor said. This surprised me. I'd never known a clergyperson to admit doubts.

"Here's one of them," he said. "If God is all-powerful and all-knowing, how is it that we also have free will? It doesn't seem like these two things should coexist. God would already know the outcome, and if He knows it, how are our actions independent of that knowing and that power?"

I agreed and quickly ran through the logic of how these ideas might be mutually exclusive — even this was a math problem to my mind, I noticed. I took out a piece of paper and a pen to draw it for him. I put an omnipotent God in a big circle, and as hard as I tried, I couldn't put people and their actions in a separate circle next to it; their actions just couldn't be independent of that kind of force, I told him. The circles wouldn't even just overlap; they would have to merge. I added that I couldn't imagine an all-powerful Creator who, in giving us choices, would also have created evil. "An all-powerful God knew torture would happen, knew the Crusades would happen; heck, God even knew that I'd be mugged, and if that's true, we are just pawns in that plan without real free will. I think evil exists to give context to the good, but if I were God, I would just let people know about evil in their imaginations and not give them the ability to act on it."

My visitor smiled and walked over to my drawings hanging behind the counter. "Did you do these?"

"Yes. I have been drawing what I see in my head for several years now. That circle is pi, and that snowflake-like design is wave-particle duality." I explained these concepts during what would turn into a three-hour conversation.

"You say you can actually see these things?" he asked at one point.

"Yes."

"This is a part of creation too, then."

"I suppose it is. To me, it is the fundamental structure of things."

"God must be quite a mathematician," he said, shaking his head and putting his hands in his pockets. "I imagine your view of the universe is much larger than my own."

I told him, "It's not universe, it's universes, plural." I explained that astronomers claim that there are about five hundred billion galaxies in addition to our celestial home — the Milky Way galaxy — and that according to string theory there are at least 10^{500} different universes. But then some physicists believe there are actually infinite universes. We started talking about the idea of parallel universes, with all possibilities existing somewhere in each their own realm. "There is a me talking with you here in one universe and at home taking a nap in another," I said.

The pastor didn't buy any merchandise that day, but he shook my hand and thanked me for expanding his view of things. I was so flattered that I didn't recoil from the touch. "I'm going to have to incorporate a lot of what you taught me today into my beliefs," he said. "My universe just got a lot bigger." And with that, he smiled and walked out the door.

Talks like that can get me through the times when I am dealing with the mundane: paperwork and inventory.

I was having a particularly busy but boring day doing just that when I saw a few high-school kids in marching-band uniforms staring at the beanbag chairs in the front window. I had purposefully put them there to entice younger customers and I saw it was working. They started spilling in, five of them flopping on the ones in the front of the store.

"These are really comfortable!" said one.

I decided to be a good sport. It was the most fun I'd probably have all day, after all. Their red, gold, and black uniforms were a striking display, as were the instruments they were carrying.

"That's because they're made with foam instead of beads," I explained. "The foam is actually a petroleum byproduct, so the price of those chairs fluctuates with the energy market."

"Cool!" said the boy holding the trombone.

More and more kids started coming through the front door and flopping down on the chairs, as well as on the mattresses and the futons. I counted forty in all.

"Isn't that a fractal?" asked one bright sixteen-year-old boy, pointing to my drawings still on display on the wall opposite him.

"Yes, it is."

"Where did you get it?"

"I drew it."

"I thought only computers could make fractals."

"Well, I can make simple ones," I explained.

"What is that circle with all the lines through it?"

"That's how I see pi."

With that, we were off and running on a discussion of pi and even relativity. I explained the concept of the Doppler effect using the different pitches of sound from a speeding car, as I had with my ex-con customer. One of the boys said, "Wow. That just changed everything!" I couldn't help but smile. We then slipped into talking about parallel universes.

One boy turned to the young woman next to him and said, "Parallel universes means that I'm the hottest guy in one universe and just perfect for you out there somewhere."

She rolled her eyes and said, "Just not here!"

I went on to explain how magnetic frequency affects our environments, only to have one boy punch another in the arm.

"Hey! Ouch!"

"That was just the magnetism — it wasn't me!" said the offender.

The tuba player asked me if I'd ever played a musical instrument. I told him I had a piano at home and had taught myself how to play.

"How did you manage that?"

"I drew staff notations with the appropriate note for each key on pieces of tape and stuck them to the keys," I explained.

"Isn't that harder than just putting the letters on them?"

"I had to see where it was on the sheet music," I offered.

"Oh."

The kids were kinetic, talking among themselves and fidgeting constantly and throwing more questions at me. Then a man walked through the front door, and I noticed they grew quiet.

"What have you done to my kids?" asked their band teacher. "I've never seen them so attentive!"

CHAPTER TWELVE

Contact

THINGS WERE BEGINNING to come back into balance, and my lopsided reality was evening out. I was inching closer to my bachelor's degree — taking two night classes every semester, as I had to continue to work full-time. Elena helped me redecorate my fortress of solitude in Hilltop into something not just livable, but downright charming. It was the first time things had felt normal in years, perhaps ever. I was very hopeful about the future and holding on to each milestone as hard as I could. *Don't go back,* I thought as I completed one exam, then one class, then two, then a semester. *Never go back. Never give up. It's not just about you now. It's for Megan and Elena too.*

But sometimes the things we hold tightest in our hands slip through them, regardless of our effort or intentions. I'd completed the equivalent of my sophomore year when a distant domino effect brought my progress to a standstill: the physical trauma of the mugging in 2002 compounded by the whiplash of a minor car accident I had had that summer finally took their toll and erupted during an entirely mundane office activity.

I was replacing one of the fifty-pound bottles in the furniture-store water cooler when I felt like I'd been hit by lightning on my left side. Seven years after the assault at the karaoke bar, I once again felt a sharp pain that brought me to my knees, and this time it left me on the floor, the water bottle missing me by inches when it fell. It was an electric, burning pain that ran from my neck down the inside of my left arm. My veins and nerves felt like power cords that were burning out in a burst of energy; just a hot, searing, burning pain. I never knew pain could be so severe. I was shaking.

There was only one thought going through my mind as I lay there, and it was not my mortality or a concern about how I was going to earn a living if I was disabled. Rather, it was *How am I going to draw and hold the ruler any longer?* I drew with my right hand, it's true, but I had to hold the ruler steady and firm with my left hand, pressing it down hard into the paper, in order to get the straightest lines and avoid errors. Sometimes I would sit like this for hours at a time, and it required some stamina to keep pressing from one side, shifting the ruler ever so precisely, then pressing down again for the next line. What if my left arm and hand no longer worked?

If a severe illness or injury does one thing, it brings your priorities into diamondlike, laser focus. It had never been clearer to me that I had to draw, that I had to create, and that if I lost that ability, I would never be myself again. I knew I had a life before this one—a full and happy one in its crazy way—but I was no longer that man and I didn't want to return to the life I'd had before I had these abilities. As a flurry of thoughts flooded my panicked mind, it was the memory of my drawings that made my heart leap into my throat.

I realized in an instant how far I'd come. Even my four years of solitude didn't feel like such a waste now that I was in school and connecting the dots between what I'd taught myself in that time and the accepted academic version of the same things. It was this realization of how far I'd come that helped me harness whatever strength I had and push myself up from the floor using my right arm. I tried to take a few steps; I was limping, I noticed. I gingerly made my way out of the store, climbed into my car, and made my way yet again to the local hospital.

I began what would be a two-year quest for wellness, through physical therapy, prescription pain medication, and, ultimately, surgery, in which a disc between the vertebrae in my neck was replaced with a titanium disc. But in the beginning, for the first two weeks after the injury, I was almost bedridden. I could barely get up to go to the bathroom. I slept a lot, and when I was not sleeping I was grimacing with the slightest movement. I remembered my dad and all those awful pains he had in his back when I was younger. I felt guilty about not realizing the true severity of such pain. At the time, I'd wondered how it could really be as bad as he said. I have such empathy for people with back injuries now. Back injuries are hidden to all but their sufferers, I realized. If you have even a little paper cut, people can see the blood. But back pain is cruel in both its severity and invisible nature. The only people who really understood what I was going through were Elena and Megan. They remained incredibly caring and helpful as I struggled.

I ultimately had to take a leave of absence from work and, worse, from Tacoma Community College. I could barely pick up a pen to do my school assignments. I could neither draw nor hold the ruler that was so crucial to my art. I was heartbroken.

The loss was enormous, even compared with the loss I felt following my mugging. It was one thing to live a carefree life of partying and lose that. It was quite another to live a life in which you were aware of what was important and were close to achieving your goals and then have that taken away from you. I sank into a deep depression.

Months passed, and I was stuck in front of the Discovery Channel and the Science Channel, attempting to keep learning in the only way I could. I watched more documentaries on black holes than I thought could possibly exist, practically memorizing Carl Sagan's speeches in the process. Sometimes I watched the same program again and again, as many times as the channel repeated it, which was a lot. It hardly mattered if I'd seen it once or three times. It was all I had. Unable to work, I drifted deeper and deeper into debt. Elena was a full-time student, and it was important to me that she not quit school to work and support us. She'd been so good to me, and I wanted to make sure my problems didn't affect her future.

There was one bright spot in this low period. I had a consultation with a neurologist, since I was considering having surgery on my neck to alleviate the pain, and I was sitting in the waiting room looking at my drawings when other patients began to ask me what they were. I took out my closely guarded portfolio of finished work and set out to explain my story and the geometry and physics that were fundamental to my art. I noticed the receptionist looking up from her work periodically until she just couldn't be silent anymore.

It turned out she had studied a lot of math herself and she understood what I was trying to get across. She came out from behind her desk to have a closer look and complimented me enthusiastically on my abilities. Moments later, I heard the buzz of the office intercom and her voice saying, "Dr. Song, please come out here. You have to meet this young man in the waiting room."

The doctor emerged and looked through my work. He smiled and said he couldn't wait to talk with me when it was my turn in his office. When that moment arrived, he asked me to tell him how I had been injured. I launched into my whole story. When I finished, he sat back and said thoughtfully, "Perhaps these abilities are due to the brain injury. You may have synesthesia and savant syndrome."

I couldn't believe the words came out of the mouth of a medical professional. It had been my private theory for so long. I told him I did think that was the case and that I'd recognized myself in the program I'd seen, years ago, on Daniel Tammet. Hearing the doctor corroborate my theory about what was going on with me buoyed my spirit all the way home. When I got inside my house and had time to reflect, I realized what I really wanted to do was celebrate by drawing something new. I was crestfallen when I couldn't move my arm well enough to hold the pencil. Weeks of further isolation and depression ensued. Then the day of the surgery arrived.

The only respites I've had from my constant visual images are the couple of times I've been completely anesthetized. That day was no different. I say completely anesthetized because at the onset of the anesthesia cocktail, I saw the images escalate. I remember feeling immobilized but seeing a circle rotating, spinning, and morphing into other shapes seconds after the IV drip was placed in my arm. Lots of other unbidden pictures also appeared, twisting to and fro, doing what they wanted. It wasn't imagination; I wasn't willing it. A little anesthesia made my impressions go crazy; a lot stamped it out. I woke up from my surgery thinking it was the only good sleep I'd had in a decade. I felt like a newborn baby and was practically giddy from the quality of the rest. I wished I slept well every night, but when I was falling asleep normally I went off to what I called fractal land. I'd see myriad shapes and colors while hypnagogic. And my dreams were often abstract and a continuation of seeing these forms; not many of my dreams were just stories or narratives. I think it was just my brain continually firing.

When I finally resurfaced — on the other end of the operation to install the titanium disc in my neck — I returned to my job at Planet Futon but couldn't afford to resume my studies. I felt the air go out of my lungs the day I did my budget to begin paying down my debt and realized that I just couldn't fit tuition into the plan. I was devastated. I felt I was making important progress in school and I was now worried that my education was lost for good. But the months of calculus and trigonometry had left their mark, and the operation had left me well enough to begin drawing again. I decided there was no more time to lose. I felt confident enough in my remaining abilities to start sharing my drawings online through a YouTube video.

There were two very important images to me at that time: one was of sine, cosine, and tangent waves and their reflections vibrating due to the speed of light making a space-time grid, and one represented fractal fusion. I'd become obsessed with the thought of the potential energy of geometry, and because these images represented that to me, I made sure I included both of them prominently in the video.

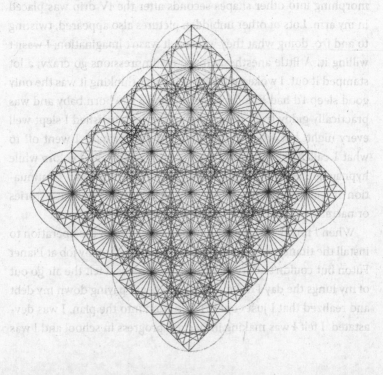

I thought of the rendering just previous as a fractal of space-time at the quantum level. If you draw a straight line and call it a Planck length and then require that all points be exactly the same distance away (or whole-number multiples of the Planck length), the only way it can be drawn is as a straight line or a lattice. The quantized structure of energy and space-time actually requires that the structure at the smallest level be a lattice. To me, this fractal has a lot of mass (and energy), as in my mind, the number of lines indicates mass. I first saw the image that inspired this drawing in the physical world when watching sunlight glistening on a lake. While one can clearly see the light points at the center of each square, the rest of it grew from my imagination as I thought about what water would be like at a specific place in time on the quantum level.

The next illustration shows particle fusion the way I imagine it.

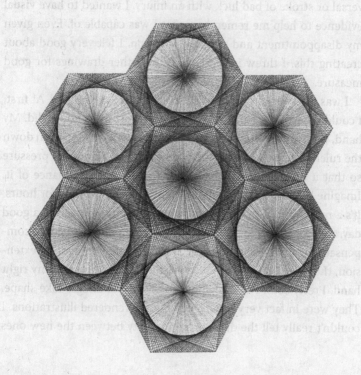

To my mind, the center hexagon is an inert iron core of a star and the six surrounding hexagons are the outer mass, collapsing toward the center (or the core) due to immense gravity. When they hit the core from all sides at nearly the exact same time, they fuse with the iron core and then rebound outward and explode as a supernova. Though this drawing shows the process as I see it, it is also a wish on my part. I dream about being involved in controlling fusion one day to create unlimited, clean energy.

From my home, I videotaped myself drawing these fractals and uploaded a time-lapse video of them onto YouTube in early November 2010. I set the video to an upbeat Hindi melody that suited them. I felt that people should know how I draw things, step by step, and this was a good way to demonstrate that. Part of me also wanted a record of these drawings in case I had another health reversal or stroke of bad luck with an injury. I wanted to have visual evidence to help me remember what I was capable of. Even given my disappointment and renewed isolation, I felt very good about creating this. I threw in a couple of my other drawings for good measure.

I was a little shaky at drawing so soon after my surgery. At first, I couldn't press the ruler into the paper as firmly as I once did. My hand, wrist, and shoulder were still so sensitive. I had to push down the ruler with my left arm with a specific, firm amount of pressure so that it didn't move, and I couldn't quite feel the balance of it. Imagine holding your arm down on a table and pushing for hours. It's a real workout from the shoulder through the wrist on a good day, and now it was too difficult. But I figured out that I could compensate for the decreased strength of my left arm and, by extension, the ruler by pressing more lightly with the pencil in my right hand. Pretty soon I was seeing some beautiful images take shape. They were in fact very steady and sharply rendered illustrations. I couldn't really tell the difference in quality between the new ones and the ones I'd completed before my most recent injury. I was feeling euphoric that I was able to practice my passion again.

In this soaring, happy state, it occurred to me as I pressed my pencil into the paper and continued drawing that I might be capturing sound in that process — kind of like pressing an old vinyl record. I was not sure how I came to this idea, but whenever euphoria strikes, I'm prone to such revelations. Actually, it's a chicken-and-egg thing; perhaps the revelation rides in just ahead of the euphoria. But it obsessed me so much that I decided to be really careful about the background sound in my environment as I created the drawings. I chose songs that were meaningful to me, like "Telephone," by Lady Gaga and Beyoncé, as if I were communicating with a scientist from a future world who would be able to pull the sound out of my impressions one day. I played other songs that were appropriate to me, like "Mother," by Pink Floyd, from the album *The Wall*. I very much related to that album. I put a YouTube video by Symphony of Science on, featuring audio by Carl Sagan and other top thinkers. It was called "We Are All Connected." The innovative videographers behind it morphed Sagan's speaking voice into song and so he sang, "We are a way for the universe to know itself," and his intellectual heir, the astrophysicist Neil deGrasse Tyson, sang, "We are all connected, to each other biologically, to the Earth chemically, and to the rest of the universe atomically."

I daydreamed for a while about the archaeologist who might one day stumble on my drawings, pick them up, and carefully brush the dust off the folder. Would the device to pull the sound out of them look like a cell phone? Would it be a wand? And what about the pi drawings that Archimedes did in ancient times? If they were scanned one day in the future, perhaps the archaeologist could pull the sound out and hear the footsteps of the Roman regiment approaching Syracuse to sack the city and behead my hero!

I snapped back to the present and put the finishing touches on my work. I turned off the audio accompaniment and decided my video was not half bad. In fact, it was really pretty provocative, I thought; I'd certainly have watched it if someone else had created it. I had a moment of doubt thinking that the people who were interested in such things were in the minority, and maybe it wouldn't ever get any recognition because there were so few people who cared about the topic. I labeled the video with the keywords *synesthesia* and *savantism*, which my doctor suspected I had and which I personally believed I had, although that was still far from being confirmed. Had I made the video even more marginal with these obscure terms? They were the only clues I had about the person I'd become, so I decided the labels must remain.

"Here goes nothing," I said as I uploaded it and sent it out into the world.

It bounced around the Internet that day and started picking up comments and interpretations and links like barnacles on a ship until finally it became a Google synesthesia alert. Alerts can be set up on Gmail accounts for practically any topic. Google cherry-picks content based in part on recommendations and then sends the results to interested people, I would learn, though I had no idea at the time that my video was spidering out across the web as I sat alone in my house.

All the way across the country, in New York City, synesthete and journalist Maureen Seaberg found the Google alert e-mail in her in box. She had set the alert up a year ago to aid in research on a book she was writing on synesthesia. It's one of several she received, but it immediately stood out.

Maureen opened the video and was floored, she told me later. She'd never seen anything like my cross-sensory drawings, though she had synesthesia herself and knew what other synesthetes experienced, and she was very active in their community, speaking at conferences and writing on the topic. She knew that while she and her friends had extraordinary visual impressions, my orderly, highly geometric shapes were a world apart. Synesthetes see photisms — colored, moving forms that appear in response to stimuli — and mine were the most complex she'd ever seen. Further, they weren't amorphous, like many photisms; they were crystalline and highly geometric.

In 1926, psychologist Heinrich Klüver became the first researcher to catalog these photisms. He did so based on studies he conducted in which people took the psychoactive drug peyote and then described the synesthetic visions they saw. Dr. Klüver noted

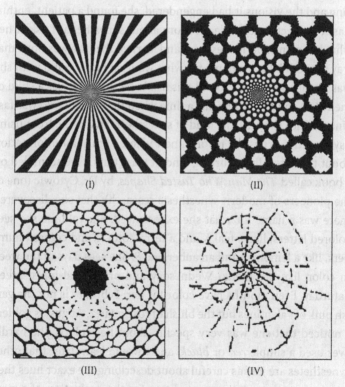

Klüver's four general form constants:
(I) tunnels, (II) spirals, (III) lattices, and (IV) cobwebs.

that most subjects reported seeing the same four geometric patterns—tunnels, spirals, lattices, and cobwebs. While some of my drawings were reminiscent of these general patterns to Maureen, they struck her as very special indeed.

My visions appeared to be several orders of magnitude more complicated and organized than those of the average synesthete, and Maureen was so excited she immediately wrote me an e-mail through YouTube under her 7synesthesia handle. It took only minutes for me to respond. I was so excited to once again discuss what I see and think that our e-mail exchange lasted almost the whole afternoon. As Maureen peppered me with questions about the mugging and the visions it had engendered, she found a patient, enthusiastic subject eager to learn more about synesthesia. I asked her what her own experiences were and learned that she was born that way but didn't have a name for what went on in her mind until she was twenty-seven. She found this ironic because she was a child of the 1960s and 1970s, like me, a time when the entire world was fascinated with the artificial kind of synesthesia that came from using psychoactive drugs but no one knew where to turn for information about the naturally occurring kind. It wasn't until she stumbled on a book called *The Man Who Tasted Shapes*, by Dr. Cytowic (one of the pioneers of modern synesthesia research), that she discovered there was a name for what she experienced. She told me she sees colored letters, like a teal *K* and a terra-cotta *R*, and colored numbers, like a lemony *2* and an aubergine *8*. She sees days of the week in color, like her indigo Wednesday and primordial-forest-green Saturday. Even months have color for her: February is not the garish pink of valentines but the blush of rose quartz. August is golden. I noticed that she was very specific about her colors. She hardly ever used a simple *red* or *black*, and I would learn later that other synesthetes are just as careful about describing the exact hues they see. In fact, the most respected test for the evaluation of synesthesia is neuroscientist and author David Eagleman's online Synesthesia Battery, and Eagleman knew not to give multiple-choice answers for colors in the battery. Instead, he installed a custom color bar so synesthetes could put their cursors over just the right shades they see.

When Maureen listened to music, she saw colored shapes, she explained. She tried her best to describe what Yo-Yo Ma playing Bach's Prelude in G Major looked like but confessed she'd really have to be a glass artisan to demonstrate the molten forms of coffee tones she saw, "like those Christmas peppermints that fold over themselves like waves." Through an online test, she told me, she'd recently discovered she had motion-to-hearing synesthesia, which meant she heard sound when she saw things move. I could hardly keep up with all the impressions. Though I'd read up on the subject on my own, I didn't realize there were so many different varieties of synesthesia. What synesthetes all have in common is some sort of blending of the senses that each person can see only him- or herself, she explained. I realized I might have stumbled upon a community I didn't even know I belonged to. Though synesthesia affects only 4 percent of the population, Maureen told me that there is a lot of interaction among synnies, as they like to be known, mostly thanks to the Internet.

A synesthete was central to the formation of the World Wide Web, interestingly enough, she said. Robert Cailliau, of Belgium, and Timothy Berners-Lee, of Great Britain, were working at the European Organization for Nuclear Research (known as CERN; the acronym originally stood for Conseil Européen pour la Recherche Nucléaire). The term *World Wide Web* came about when Berners-Lee suggested it and Cailliau agreed because his synesthetic *W* was dark green, his favorite color! As a result of the web, she said, there are both formal organizations and loosely associated people on social media today all finding one another and comparing sensory impressions. I could see why those people might want to be in touch, as I was enjoying the shorthand Maureen and I were using in our e-mails. She had many questions and much information to share, but she got what I was saying more quickly than most nonsynesthetes because of the common ground we had. Perhaps most important, she took me at my word when I described what I saw. Since she had similar experiences, she believed me unquestioningly. She knew it was a thing.

Elena and I were planning to fly to New York City, two weeks from the day I uploaded the video, while on our way to Boston to meet with planetarium makers who wanted me to consult on a project. They had found me through a mutual friend on Facebook and needed my advice on teaching fractal geometry to children in their presentation. I told Maureen, and she asked to meet with us while we were in her hometown of New York City. We exchanged phone numbers and regular e-mails, and when the day arrived we met for a casual lunch and the three of us got to know one another. I could tell she recognized the enormous scope of my experiences and the mysteries left in their wake. And she had a great day planned for me. After lunch we would meet with a literary agent and a filmmaker and then make our way to the United Nations, where a leader in the synesthesia community, Patricia Lynne Duffy, worked as an editor and trainer and had arranged a full tour for me! Duffy, the author of *Blue Cats and Chartreuse Kittens: How Synesthetes Color Their Worlds*, the first book about synesthesia by a synesthete, was the cofounder of a group called the American Synesthesia Association (ASA) and a big advocate for research into our shared abilities. Duffy saw colored numbers and letters and had a form of synesthesia I can't even imagine: spatial sequence, in which the alphabet rose upward, left to right, when she visualized it, each letter always occupying a specific point in space. She was an expert in literary synesthesia as well, versed in the writing of both confirmed synesthetes and nonsynesthetes who created fiction with synesthetic characters. Her knowledge was encyclopedic, and I never would have guessed there were so many synesthete authors as well as nonsynesthete authors who find the ability so interesting that they give it to their characters in fiction. We also talked about a number of high-profile synesthetes who were coming out of the closet, like Billy Joel, Pharrell Williams, Geoffrey Rush, Tilda Swinton, Orhan Pamuk, and Itzhak Perlman, some of whom confessed their abilities for the first time ever to Maureen. She liked to out them, with their permission, to help erase the stigma of the syndrome. Duffy was a warm and welcoming woman, and she talked about everything from the organization of the United Nations to the stories behind the beautiful art lining the hallways. She even took my picture in the General Assembly, a photo I still treasure. She later said to Maureen, "It was such a fascinating talk and Jason was so genuine. I could see he was taking in the beauty of something immense and newly discovered. It was very touching." By the time Maureen and I broke for dinner, I felt like it was a pretty great thing to be part of the community of synesthetes; it was actually an asset to count myself among these very creative and interesting people. I noticed I didn't feel so lonely.

A new friendship formed, and in the coming days, Maureen reached out in a white heat to other synesthetes and neuroscientists on my behalf, spreading the word about my case and carving out a path for me to continue my education. She was about to moderate a synesthesia panel at a Toward a Science of Consciousness conference in Stockholm, and she invited me to present my case and my theories. I was happy to learn Duffy would also be there. Maureen contacted another participant of the conference, Berit Brogaard — a philosopher who studied cognitive neuroscience, philosophy of mind, and philosophy of language — to see if she would study me. Dr. Brogaard was a professor of philosophy at the University of Missouri in St. Louis and the director of the Brogaard Lab for Multisensory Research, which was affiliated with a top laboratory in Helsinki, Finland. Brogaard was immediately intrigued. After my week at the conference in Stockholm, I would fly to the lab in Helsinki. Brogaard had scheduled a series of tests for me at the Brain Research Unit, Low Temperature Laboratory (since renamed the O. V. Lounasmaa Laboratory), at Aalto University. A team of scientists would meet us there. Maybe I would finally get a firm diagnosis! Like Maureen, Dr. Brogaard was convinced I was a special case due to the sudden onset of my abilities after my injury. Perhaps it was also because, as I learned later, she herself had pain-to-color synesthesia and thought of pain as a purple mountain. She saw it with her own eyes, so she believed me when I told her what I saw. The synesthetes I was meeting were all receptive to me and didn't find my impressions the least bit strange.

I was almost back to the feeling I had had when I left for Russia for the first time: I hadn't been out of my house much at all for months, and suddenly I was planning to go halfway around the world to talk about myself and finally get the proper tests I hadn't had access to or the money for before. I began to wonder how my back would fare on the long flight to Europe, and I worried I wouldn't even be able to stand up to exit the aircraft, much less stand on a stage and tell my story. I wanted the opportunity to participate in the conference and take the diagnostic tests so badly that I expressed nothing but enthusiasm, though. I prepared a strap and pillow to use on the plane that would keep my head in place so I wouldn't hurt myself if I fell asleep. I started to deliberate which drawings to include in the talk and what to say.

I left New York feeling hopeful and validated. Meeting my first synesthetes removed a lot of the doubts I had had about myself. I gained more confidence in my abilities from that meeting and was energized to do even more with my drawings.

Maureen shared with me the written mission statement of the Center for Consciousness Studies — which is based at the University of Arizona in Tucson, though its conferences take place at various sites around the globe — so I would have a better sense of the concept behind the conferences.

I learned that the science of human consciousness remains poorly understood. The dominance of behaviorism in psychology that stamped out interest in the once-popular topic of synesthesia also hurt the study of consciousness, but curiosity about the science behind both topics has risen recently. The University of Arizona has been key in these developments. The first Toward a Science of Consciousness conference, which took place in Tucson in 1994, was a landmark event. The conference has been held each year since then in locations around the world.

It sounded like just the place to tell my story publicly for the first time. Maureen said that mind-body guru Deepak Chopra, physicist and author Leonard Mlodinow, neuropsychiatrist Peter Fenwick, and mathematical physicist Sir Roger Penrose would be present — all giants in the realms of philosophy, neuroscience, mathematics, or quantum physics. I couldn't believe I was being transported from a futon store in Tacoma into their company.

For my presentation, I would describe my injury and subsequent impressions as well as display and explain my geometric drawings. I decided to try to record this event and began seeking videographers who might want to travel with me. After interviewing several candidates, I settled on the affable Paul Synowiec. His work samples were very impressive, and, just as important, he was a very easygoing person able to get along with me from the start.

CHAPTER THIRTEEN

Savant and Yogi?

THOUGH I WAS happy and inspired by my trip to New York, the flight back to Tacoma turned out to be a difficult one for me physically. I fidgeted the entire six hours to relieve aches and pains and was incredibly stiff and sore upon arrival. With the trip to Stockholm only a few months away, I worried that I'd have an even more difficult time during my next flight. My doctor recommended a pain-management clinic and I signed up immediately.

Attending the clinic was like a job; it required me to go five days a week for eight hours a day for two months. On the menu of services were meditation, exercise, group therapy, and regular medical consultations with a team of doctors. The meditation and group therapy were new experiences for me, and I was somewhat nervous about trying them. I found myself once again taking time off from the futon store. I was pretty useless there anyway, as I was in so much pain.

Elena was really concerned about me during this time. She told me she thought the words *pain-management clinic* sounded really awful and she was worried that I needed something so serious. But we thought I should try it, as nothing else was making me better.

"I want you to imagine your whole body relaxing," said our soft-spoken meditation leader on the first day; I was lying flat on a mat on the floor. "Breathe in, breathe out, from your belly to your chest; deep, deep breaths."

I watched as not only my chest but also my stomach rose. It was incredible how much more air I could get in my lungs that way.

"Now imagine the tips of your fingers relaxing, feel it through your wrists; now your elbows . . . Continue to breathe in and breathe out from your stomach. Feel the relaxation extend to your shoulders."

I felt my arms turn to Jell-O. I had never once in my life stopped so completely to focus on relaxing. It felt amazing.

"Now pause and relax everything some more, take it further."

I didn't think it was possible to go even more limp and more re-laxed, but I followed the instruction and found myself practically sinking into the hardwood floor beneath me.

For five to ten minutes, I felt a weird but totally pleasant and warm state of well-being. When we rose slowly from the mats at the end of the exercise, my pain was lessened. It was a watershed moment for me. I never knew I had this ability inside me. I'd been so frenetic for years, and stillness had been the furthest thing from my mind. Even in my years of isolation in my home, my mind had been racing. No one was more surprised than me that there was ac-tually something to this meditation practice. Perhaps my mind re-ally could help heal my body, I thought.

I became more practiced at meditation in the coming days and weeks, and the instructor asked me to participate in a little experi-ment. I was game. He hooked me up to some electrodes and tested my ability to self-modulate. He had me look at an electronic moni-tor as sine wave after sine wave went by like a series of hills on a cross-country drive. I tried to make the apex of each wave as round as possible through regular, deep breathing and focused attention.

"Okay, I've got this!" I said excitedly at one point, noticing how I was able to help form a beautiful, symmetrical wave every ten seconds.

The instructor next took my pulse and blood pressure. I'd succeeded in lowering both considerably in our session. He was amazed to learn the temperature of my skin had gone up about six or seven degrees — something he'd never recorded a person doing on a first try before, he said.

"You're really good at this for a beginner, Jason — bravo!" he remarked. "Now, make sure you continue to practice at home."

When we were finished I walked over to the chalkboard in the room and drew a blood vessel — a cylinder, really — for the instructor to consider. I drew cross sections of it in a subsequent rendering and explained how my temperature was raised due to increased blood flow and surface area in my vessels.

"That's right!" said the instructor.

"Even our bodies come down to geometry," I said with a smile as I turned to leave.

I was really fascinated by this practice and so convinced of its healing effects that I started telling friends and relatives that it should be taught to every human being, everywhere. In fact, I said, I believed that young children should learn this in school. It was as important as any other skill we could acquire in life. I bet it would have a positive effect on global relations if everyone would take the time to meditate each day.

While meditating at home once, I found myself thinking of a pentagon, like the one I'd seen on my late stepfather's uniform. I started to draw it, exploring its inner space with additional lines and angles according to things I was now seeing in my mind's eye, inspired by the initial shape. Only this time, instead of the image being extremely beautiful and two-dimensional, it was much more beautiful and seemed to appear in three dimensions. I couldn't believe my eyes. It was as though I had just stepped from a gray Kansas plain into the Technicolor land of Oz.

I sat there exploring this development for some time. I noticed I could shift my attention and throw the shapes out from my mind's eye into space around me so that I was standing amid them. Then I could move my attention toward them and float over them, under them, even behind them, projecting my awareness out into space. It was so cool. I stared at it and saw how it had depth for the first time, and I was transfixed. Some lines appeared to be behind other ones instead of flat as they had before. I'd never seen anything so stunning.

I arrived early to the pain-management clinic the next day just to report this to my instructor. "Perhaps because of your practice, your mind is refining these images even further," he said, delighted.

I continued to work on my first 3-D drawing in celebration of

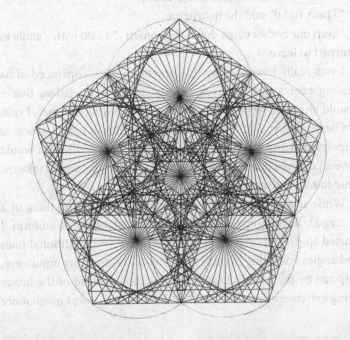

this development. The image, which I titled "Quantum Star," came to me as I explored the inner spaces of a pentagon.

I told Maureen about this development and she thought it was so significant she put me in touch with another conference participant I would be presenting with in Stockholm, the medical anthropologist William C. Bushell, then the director of East-West Research for Tibet House in New York. The Harvard- and MIT-trained researcher had spent thirty years documenting the health benefits of meditation and had heard about all sorts of experiences, many of them from really adept yogis and lamas from the Indo-Tibetan tradition. At Tibet House, Dr. Bushell worked with the Columbia professor Robert Thurman, an Indo-Tibetan studies scholar who also happened to be the actress Uma Thurman's father. Together, the researchers ran their own conferences featuring His Holiness the Dalai Lama and other great meditation experts.

I still wondered if what I was seeing was tied to some fundamental fabric of things. Could I be seeing the hidden structure of what's all around us at some beyond-microscopic level?

"It is indeed possible to see things at the quantum level of the photon," Dr. Bushell explained to me, noting cutting-edge biological research on the human retina that proved humans could detect light at its quantum-mechanical limits, something no artificial detection device could surpass. He cited the work of Princeton biophysicist William Bialek.

"Our eyes are actually that subtle, but we don't all have access to it at a conscious level. Adept meditators report some of the things you are seeing, so it may be tied to meditation somehow." Dr. Bushell referred me to scientific papers backing up what he told me, and he himself had published papers connecting this amazing discovery to things advanced meditators said about what they saw in darkened environments. As far back as 1998, University of Washington professor Fred Rieke and Stanford neurobiologist Denis Baylor had written, in *Reviews of Modern Physics,* that our eyes were "nearly perfect photon counters."

This made me wonder: if the human eye is equipped to see at the quantum level, why doesn't everybody see what I see? I went back to brain science to look for answers. Our brains are very, very busy — each one processing millions of bits of visual information with each passing second. Experts have long believed that the brain filters out the vast majority of this incoming raw data. Did this mean that other people's eyes were receiving the same visual input mine did, but their brains were just weeding it out like some sort of visual spam? It made me wish I could tell people how to switch off the brain's filter so they could see what I see, because it definitely isn't spam.

The more I talked with Dr. Bushell, the more I thought that meditation might be one way for people to remove those filters. According to Bushell's extensive research, people who meditate regularly may be able to enhance the way their visual systems work, which might allow them to see things in nature that are hidden from non-meditators. I had been seeing the hidden fabric of the world in all those geometric shapes already; Dr. Bushell explained that meditation might have something to do with the sudden blossoming of my synesthesia from two dimensions to three.

The medical anthropologist believed synesthetes had extraordinary doorways to perception and said that even the great Japanese Zen master Dōgen had written of synesthesia being present at enlightenment. Dr. Bushell had told Maureen in a previous interview, "Synesthesia may not only be associated with the highest spiritual states, it may be *necessary* for them." I had never really thought about the concept of enlightenment before, but the more I learned about it, the more what Dr. Bushell was saying made sense to me. Some of the terms I came across in my research on enlightenment were *awakening, self-awareness,* and *understanding the connected-*

ness of everything. I could see how synesthetes, with their blended senses, might be more in tune with these things.

When I told Dr. Bushell about the pain relief I'd experienced after meditating, he wasn't surprised at all. In fact, he told me that when it comes to relieving pain, scientific evidence shows that meditation and hypnosis can be just as effective as opioids — the most powerful pharmacological treatment. He said that brain-imaging studies showed how it works. One study that was especially encouraging to me was a joint effort between the University of California, Irvine, and the Institute for Natural Medicine and Prevention. They used fMRI brain scans to test the response to pain in twelve long-term meditators and twelve nonmeditators. Compared to the nonmeditators, the meditators showed up to 50 percent less activity in areas of the brain associated with pain response. But what was really cool was that after the nonmeditators spent five months learning how to meditate, their scans showed up to 50 percent reduced activity in the brain's pain centers compared to their first test.

Equally exciting to me was learning that the practice also reduced symptoms associated with PTSD. One study that appeared in *Military Medicine* found that veterans returning from Iraq and Afghanistan who practiced meditating for just eight weeks reduced their PTSD symptoms by 50 percent. If it was that helpful for Marines returning from war zones, then it just might be helpful for me too.

To get the maximum benefit from meditation, however, I needed to learn how to relax and clear my mind, because I couldn't stop the images I saw, even with my eyes closed. What a surprise to hear Dr. Bushell say that the stereotypical notion of meditation as a clearing of the mind or a lack of thought isn't the only way to do it. Apparently, some people practice types of meditation specifically designed to develop mental imagery. I was glad I didn't have to worry that I always needed to see a black screen when I closed my eyes for my meditation to be effective.

From everything I had told Dr. Bushell, he said he thought that something extraordinary was going on with my skill at concentrating, something he referred to as yogic ability. He said that savants have an enormous ability to focus, and he thought that my success at self-regulating my blood pressure, heart rate, and skin temperature signaled a high aptitude for meditation. I had to agree. I'd never before been able to sit still and ponder things. And what about the four years I'd spent holed up in my home just thinking?

He told me that even Einstein and Newton practiced this sort of isolation, meditating on a problem. I couldn't believe that my behavior mirrored that of my scientific heroes, not to mention that of some of the top meditators of the world. Talking with Dr. Bushell confirmed for me I was on the right path with this new practice in my life.

In Stockholm I got to meet Dr. Bushell in person as well as his collaborator Neil Theise, a physician, stem-cell researcher, synesthete, and Zen student for twenty-five years. Their double-act presentation for Maureen's synesthesia workshop at the consciousness meeting and the discussions in the group that followed expanded on many of these themes of meditation and consciousness. I could hardly wait to learn more about how it all might apply to me.

I would later get to talk with Dr. Theise about how I fit into the wider theme of the conference: that it was about not only biology but also consciousness and its various forms. He talked to me about the self-organizing nature of the universe, the idea that the world self-assembles from the smallest Planck scale all the way up through the everyday world to the vast, cosmic scale. He said that according to long-accepted theories, the smallest things — whether they were strings or particles or something else — were thought to bubble into existence out of a so-called quantum foam. We can thank Nobel Prize–winning physicist John Archibald Wheeler for this concept of a sort of bubbling foam of matter, antimatter, and space-time itself. The geometry at this level, as Dr. Theise pointed out, is distorted, and there are no smooth edges.

No smooth edges? Not even at the tiniest level? Upon learning this, I could hardly contain my excitement. In my mind, this validated not only my belief that fractal geometry and its ability to measure roughness is profoundly important but also my belief that a circle has no smooth curvature when viewed at the smallest scale.

Dr. Theise went on to say that most of this infinitesimally small stuff immediately self-destructs and vanishes, but some of it interacts to "self-assemble into subatomic particles and then into atoms, into molecules, all the way on up to form our bodies, stars and planets, galaxies." Once again, this made me think of all the fractals I see throughout the universe, and I felt like I must have been on to something when I thought that everything and everyone is a reflection of the same repetitive structure.

But then the stem-cell researcher ventured into philosophical territory that I hadn't even begun to consider. If everything is self-assembling from quantum foam that comes from nothing, "then what is this nothing out of which everything arises?" he asked. Dr. Theise told me how one perspective, based equally on contemporary Western philosophy and first-person reports from Dr. Bushell's adept meditators, proposes that this nothingness is the mind itself — and that *everything* is mind.

Up until this point in my research into my condition, I had been learning how brain chemistry determines what happens in our minds. What Dr. Theise was saying flipped that around, implying that the mind cannot be explained by just looking at the brain, but rather that the mind itself may be fundamental — that the physical universe may arise from the mind.

In addition to introducing me to a new way to look at the mind, Dr. Theise also pointed me to a different theory on synesthesia. Dr. Theise himself has the spatial-sequence form of synesthesia, seeing his time units out in space around him. So far, I had found lots of research claiming that synesthesia develops when wires in the brain get crossed. But Dr. Theise suggested that it might go deeper than that. In his view, the mind or consciousness underlies all of existence, and the brain is merely filtering out everything that isn't necessary for daily functioning. He likened it to the way you can tune in to a specific radio station. There are millions of radio signals out there, but the radio is able to filter through them all to zero in on the one you want to hear. "When a radio can't be tuned," he said, "it's not actually transmitting too little information, it's transmitting *too much* information. The overlapping, multiple signals collide in our ears. Similarly, in the deeper mind accessed by the meditator, in the mind that is as yet unfiltered by the brain for everyday functioning, there is no separation of one sense or another."

One thing Dr. Theise told me that really surprised me was that some people think that all babies are synesthetic and that this innate blending of the senses is filtered out as the brain develops. This made me think of some articles I had come across in my research showing that, compared to adults, two- and three-year-olds have twice as many connections, called synapses, in the brain. Scientists say that these extra connections get weeded out through childhood and adolescence. So maybe it was true. Maybe we are all born synesthetes, but most of us lose the gift as our brains develop.

Dr. Theise then described his own experiences with meditation with a tidbit from left field that brought me back to Newton and Einstein: "Without exception, all my best research ideas — the kind that I *know* are right even before I confirm them experimentally — have come to me while I was meditating."

Although my conversations with Dr. Bushell and Dr. Theise provided a lot of insight, I felt like I had more questions than ever. The more I learned, the more I realized how much I didn't know. In my quest to discover what was happening in my brain and how I fit into the world at large, I was beginning to think that I might have to open my mind to a variety of different theories about how the universe really works.

Word was starting to get around about me within this community. Even a top Tibetan lama being studied at New York University by Dr. Bushell and the director of the contemplative Neuroscience Lab at NYU, Zoran Josipovic, had heard of me. A political refugee who had apparently cured his own gangrene by using a form of meditation known as *tsa lung,* he was being examined in brain-scan machines while meditating. Phakyab Rinpoche is believed to be a living master of the *tsa lung* discipline. Its adherents visualize moving a purifying air through the channels of the body to cleanse and heal.

Rinpoche sent a message to me and said that had I not suffered through the attack and all the subsequent pain involved, I might never have achieved the ability to meditate so effectively. And I certainly might not have the empathy for others that I now had.

"Sickness is bad, but it made you focus and be strong. If something negative hadn't happened, you wouldn't have these positives. It is a gift."

He suggested that when I meditated I shouldn't just close my eyes. Rather, he wanted me to concentrate and meditate on a purifying wind flowing through all the channels of my body, clearing out disease. In addition, I might imagine a single pebble being dropped in a puddle and radiating out to cleanse my body from within.

I was very appreciative that this lama had taken an interest in me. He had been through excruciating pain like me and had used the power of his own mind to heal himself. It helped me to forge on. And when I experienced new pain or tremors, I found myself imagining the wind or the pebble. It continues to be helpful to me and lessens my pain and anxiety.

Another aspect of the pain-management clinic that I was learning to enjoy was the gym. I hadn't worked out for years but I was now lifting weights and using the treadmill available at the center.

A big hurdle for me was getting past the idea that if I did something that hurt, like lifting weights, I was further damaging myself. The therapists explained that this was a common misconception among people who've been badly injured. Avoiding weight-lifting might lead to muscle atrophy, bone-density loss, and a lack of conditioning, and that was what would really hurt me in the long run, they said.

Though I was making great progress in the clinic's program, the group-therapy sessions remained a challenge. Before the sessions, I worried about how hard it would be for me and the other participants to reveal the details of our private lives. One day, I arrived at eight o'clock to do my morning stretches before the meeting, and I was already starting to feel anxious. I knew it was going to be a very emotional day for all of us, delving into our difficult histories and speaking publicly about them.

The group convened, and our leader encouraged us to share what was on our minds. The patients began to tell their stories, one by one. One man talked about how exhausted he was living with chronic pain and how it distracted him from his life goals, and I felt myself physically tense up because I so related to him. He added that the sexist myth that men should always be strong and able made him feel doubly bad. I realized I was beginning to feel both his discomfort and my own as I listened.

Then a hard-looking young woman named Sunny began to speak. I had learned from our previous conversations that she used to be in a gang but had left that life behind. Just as she was getting her life back together, she suffered a back injury.

"I've been a tough, strong girl my whole life," she said. "But now it's so bad having people just look at me and unable to see what's wrong with me and still expecting me to work like before. . . . People are treating me like I'm a wimp or lazy and don't want to work. They say, 'Oh, everyone gets a sore back once in a while.'"

I didn't realize it, but tears were running down my face as she said this. I felt sorry for her and was reminded of my own situation with family, friends, and colleagues who still expected me to lift heavy things at the store all day long as I had for years and who treated me like I was complaining for no reason. Most of all, I just thought of my chronic pain and whether I would have to live this way for the rest of my life.

I looked up at my instructor and realized she was staring at me. Then I felt the moisture on my face. I pointed to the door, asking to leave. She nodded.

I went across the hall to an empty office, sat in a chair, and thought about Sunny. She had been kind to me earlier, listening to my whole life story. Tough as she was, she hugged me at the time and said, "I ain't never known nobody like you before, Jason." I felt bad for her right now, and bad for the other people who spoke. And then I realized how much I'd been suffering for years and years. I started really bawling, just howling. I hadn't cried that hard since my son died. And then I remembered him and I let out a wail.

I couldn't stop. All the tears I had not shed about the mugging poured out of me. So did the anger and sadness over my brother's and stepfather's deaths. I realized I'd never properly mourned any of these losses. Now they were all hitting me simultaneously in a tsunami of pain.

My body was shaking and I felt like I needed to run but I didn't know where I should go. I could barely catch my breath as the now silent sobbing came in waves and my lungs heaved. My whole body alternately lurched and cramped. I could barely sit up in the chair.

A doctor came in and tried to comfort me but I was inconsolable. I couldn't speak when she asked me what was wrong. I just shook my head vigorously to indicate I couldn't even talk. She'd been kind to me in the past and had asked about my drawings.

I barely noticed that she'd walked across the room to the windows. Then I heard her say:

"Jason, how many windows can you count on that building facade across the street?"

I looked up.

With that, I took a big gulp of air as though I'd just surfaced from an ocean dive.

"There are twelve."

"Great," she said. "How many panes are there in each window?"

My shoulders were still heaving uncontrollably but I counted them and saw there were eight in each window and I managed to say that aloud too.

The doctor continued to engage me with questions about things outside the window: "How many branches are on the tree? Is it moving left or right in the wind?" and I was able to answer.

She handed me a paper and a pen and asked me to draw her something. I asked for a ruler and was on my way. I sat like this for a very long time until I'd made a pi diagram.

She put her hand on my shoulder when I gave it to her and she smiled.

What just happened? I wondered. I was exhausted — I felt like I'd just run fifteen miles. The staff kept me after hours and ordered me a cab because they didn't want me to drive home alone. The doctor gave me a Valium to take when I got home so I could sleep, but I just lay in my bed meditating and had no trouble falling into a deep slumber within minutes.

The next day the staff told me it was the worst panic attack they had ever seen. The doctor explained that the reason she asked me to begin counting things was to shut down the pain gateway neurologically. I asked her to explain.

"Constant pain like you have produces the chemicals that cause panic attacks to be released in your body pretty regularly," she began. "You probably have had stomach problems as a result of this too."

She went on to explain that there was a neurological gateway for pain, which I had to guard diligently. The basic concept, she said, was that both pain and pleasure signals traveled via nerve fibers in the spinal cord to the brain, but only so many signals at one time could make it through the gateway and into the brain. The idea was to flood the brain with pleasant feelings so the pain signals couldn't get through. One way to do that was to rub my left arm when it hurt. What actually happened when I did this, the doctor said, was that the sensations from the rubbing kept some of the pain signals from getting through to my brain. It worked for emotions as well, and the doctor suggested I try distracting myself when I was in pain emotionally.

By asking me to count the windows and panes and other objects, she had been trying to distract me from the overwhelming thoughts making me panic and alter the chemistry of my brain. And it worked!

"We nearly called 911, and if you hadn't responded, we would have," she admitted. "We were afraid you were going to have a seizure."

I was not political about many things but I now felt very strongly about the need for pain management for people everywhere. I was comforted to learn that there's a global organization called the International Association for the Study of Pain (IASP) that's dedicated to promoting research on chronic pain, increasing knowledge about it, and improving treatment. The group has called for the relief of pain to be a human right. I couldn't agree more. I felt some relief just knowing that there are people out there who understood.

People couldn't or wouldn't stop asking me to do the things I could no longer do, but I was learning to manage my response to their ignorance much better now. I reflected sometimes on my breakdown at the clinic and realized it was the most intense wave of anguish I'd ever felt. It was just raw sadness built up for so long for so many reasons, compounded by the profound empathy I was feeling for the other people in my class and multiplied by all the people living around the world whose suffering was apparent to me at that moment. It was all my pain amplified by all their pain.

When the pain-management clinic was over, I was saddened, though my fellow patients and I promised to keep in touch. When I left, the staff gave me the yoga mat I'd come to love so I could use it at home, and another curious gift — a simple green dot sticker.

"What's this?" I asked.

"Place it somewhere you'll always see it," said a staffer as he shook my hand in farewell. "And when you look at it, remind yourself to breathe deeply and relax."

The green dot decorates the rearview mirror of my car to this day.

It's All Relative

S OMETIMES I PICTURED my brain as a cloud producing a multitude of thunderbolts—the lightning radiating throughout my nervous system. These bolts from the blue could be moments of pure inspiration some would call genius. Other times, the lightning storm just rattled my body.

I was just beginning to feel hopeful again when it started once more: fasciculations, from my tongue to my toes. Like little earthquakes all over me, hundreds of them a day, they reminded me nearly constantly that my brain was still experiencing a kind of thunderstorm.

This had been going on for years, since right after the mugging, but lately it had become more pronounced.

The most frequent tremor I experienced was in my upper left thigh, just below where I used to keep my cell phone in my pocket. Now I couldn't keep my phone there because I'd likely ignore it, thinking it was my condition. Friends told me they also sometimes heard phantom phone rings or felt vibrations in the places where they usually kept their phones. I found it fascinating that a similar phenomenon was affecting them (it's known by various inventive terms, such as *ringxiety, hypovibrochondria,* and *faux-cell-alarm*), but in my case, the sensation could occur anywhere on my body—not just where I kept my phone—and never with disembodied sounds, like my friends reported. Both conditions are mysterious and not yet well understood, though mine is neurological, and *ringxiety* may be either neurological or psychiatric in nature. I was told there was nothing doctors could prescribe for my condition. I would just have to tolerate it. It was not painful; just annoying.

I worked on distracting myself when it happened, remembering to breathe from my stomach to draw in more breath and relax, and I did my best to ignore it. It would have driven me crazy if I acknowledged it fully every time—it was as if someone were poking me, again and again and again.

One thing the doctors did tell me is that in most cases, the symptoms can be greatly reduced by lowering overall daily stress. Stress can wreak havoc on your muscles and nerves, they told me, due to a rush of hormones and increased blood flow. I would need to exercise, get plenty of sleep, continue with my meditation practice, and lower my caffeine intake.

Adrenaline plays the most central role in creating the tremors—*adrenaline* is another name for the hormone epinephrine, which is released in response to any kind of stress. It serves to increase cardiorespiratory abilities, making it easier to fight or flee.

I'd been exercising again, and that might have been contributing to my tremors. Exercise caused higher adrenaline levels in the body, the doctors said. Untrained people will have a greater rush of the hormone than athletes. I didn't want to stop exercising, so I just had to hope the tremors would improve along with my conditioning level.

Little is known about the origins of fasciculations; no one is sure if they're brain-based or muscle-based, but the fact that they started so soon after my head trauma made me believe they came from the brain. I wondered if the seat of this phenomenon could be the parietal lobe — the very same area that likely gave me conscious awareness of the processes of math. It remained to be seen what that part of my brain looked like in depth; I hoped the testing in Helsinki after the Stockholm conference would give me some answers.

As exhausting as my challenges were, and as sad as they made me, I continued to try to move ahead. Sometimes my life felt like one step forward and two steps back. I regained my ability to draw — a giant leap forward — then had the biggest panic attack anyone had ever seen at the pain-management clinic. Must I forever push the boulder up the hill only to watch it roll back down and then have to begin again?

I knew that I was much more fortunate than most savants, many of whom struggle with overwhelming disabilities; some, like the sculptor Alonzo Clemons, are barely able to form sentences. The man on whom *Rain Man* was based, Kim Peek, couldn't even tie his own shoes. My tradeoffs might not have been as severe, but they were legion. Some days they felt like death by a thousand paper cuts — tiny but really annoying little wounds, sharp as knives.

Though my muscle twitches were ever present and distracting, they were not the worst of my tradeoffs. The majority of the unpleasant side effects of becoming a savant had to do with my OCD. It thickened the atmosphere around me; made it seem as if I were moving through molasses. I used to move through life like quicksilver, darting from one experience to the next, and now it was like my feet were in cement. When I climbed stairs, I had to count the steps; when I brushed my teeth, the brush had to go under the water a specific number of times; when someone shook my hand, I practically had to bathe in antibacterial lotion afterward. I even counted the waves of my muscle twitches when I was unable to ignore them. All of the things most people do in the course of a day without even noticing—insignificant little actions—stopped me cold. Everything felt so damn slow, despite a mind, or part of a mind, that moved faster through intellectual pursuits than ever before. It was very frustrating. The most curious thing about it was that I was totally aware of it and desperately wanted to change it but was powerless to do so.

A couple of weeks out of the clinic, I hit a wall. All of the physical and emotional burdens were adding up to a funk that I knew I must finally face—it was depression. I'd battled it after the mugging and had overcome it, but it was back, fogging up the windshield of my mind. I spent more time now in sadness and found it harder and harder to recover. The panic attack in the clinic made me realize things were getting to me deeply and I must face the fact that my new life didn't come without costs.

Perhaps the biggest side effect of my depression was that I was unable to handle confrontation at the store. There were plenty of opportunities for conflict, from the colorful customers to the sales and delivery staff. I found myself withdrawing and needing more and more time on my own. But it was more than that—I was withdrawing from even benign encounters now. Only a few months after meeting Maureen in New York and only a few weeks before the Stockholm conference, I stopped returning Maureen's calls and e-mails. I felt bad about it, especially when she was so intent on helping me. I didn't know if anyone understood, but despite my general empathy and sympathy for other people, I was closing off. The walls were going up around me. I made time for Elena and Megan and not much else. I know they were worried about me. And I worried and still worry a lot about them. Megan had been brought to tears a couple of times by my health problems. I began to think that it must be weird living with me. I knew they loved me, and I loved them. But I also knew it was hard for them and tiring to hear about my issues all the time — both the euphoric math monologues and the downtimes when I didn't feel well. In fact, I'd begun to make it a point to talk less about these things around them, even though I couldn't help myself a lot of the time.

One night when I was lying in bed, I began to think about how much easier it would be to just be dead. I was alarmed by this thought. I'd never felt this way before. How could this be happening now, when I was on the verge of a breakthrough with the upcoming conference and diagnostic testing? I even thought about using the gun I usually took with me to the store for self-defense. It was as though I had two minds: one that wanted to harm me and one that wanted to protect me. When I started thinking about the gun, I realized I needed help and went to the emergency room at the local hospital, and they kept me for six hours. Once they were convinced I was past the worst of it, they released me. I took the bullets out of my gun and put them in one end of the house; the gun with its empty chamber I put in a safe in the opposite end of the house. I didn't want to act on this thought that bubbled up, and I was not taking any chances. The walk I would have to take from one end of the house to the other might be enough time for the bad thoughts to dissipate. I was shocked and ashamed that it had come to this sort of thinking.

At this point, I began therapy. The trip to the ER was the last straw. I had insurance for the first time in years and could finally seek some help. My doctor put me on the antidepressant Zoloft. Three days after starting it, I woke in the middle of the night. I was hyperventilating and having a full-out panic attack again. I just couldn't catch my breath and I was sweating profusely. I paced the floors, trying to walk it out, as though it were only additional energy and I could just burn it off. Not wanting a six-hour stay in the emergency room again, I decided to wait it out. It felt like an eternity until my doctor's office opened at nine. He told me this could possibly be a side effect of the medicine. He weaned me off the pills and we tried the antianxiety medicine Xanax as well as talk therapy for a while instead. I began to feel more stable.

I learned that the pain medications I had been on could also have depressive side effects, so I had my doctor wean me off Dilaudid. Dilaudid is a very strong opioid drug and terribly addictive. It's a derivative of morphine, and it's a narcotic. They had put me on morphine in the hospital but I immediately suffered morphine headaches and needed a change. The withdrawal from Dilaudid was one thousand times harder than when I gave up chewing tobacco years ago. I had the worst withdrawal symptoms, from bowel problems to the shakes. My skin burned like I was on fire then switched to freezing. I would sweat and simultaneously feel like there were icicles hanging off me, the hot-and-cold cycles were so rapid.

I meditated regularly to lessen the side effects and headed back to my computer to find out if my depression could have anything to do with my brain injury. A few clicks on my keyboard and I quickly realized that depression is one of the most common symptoms of TBI. In fact, some statistics show that more than half of all TBI survivors develop the mood disorder within the first year, and nearly two-thirds have it within seven years. Somehow, I had made it almost ten years before falling into its clutches, but I learned that, like all TBI survivors, I would be at increased risk for depression for the rest of my life. According to some reports, I was ten times more likely to have it at some point during my lifetime than a person without a brain injury.

Why is depression so common after a brain injury? I wondered. Researchers are still trying to figure it out, but they've suggested many possibilities. In some people, there may be injuries to parts of the brain involved in mood stability. Other times, the depression may not be directly related to the damage to the brain. Instead, it may be connected to some of the unpleasant side effects that can come with TBI: changes in cognitive function, inability to work, or physical pain.

I didn't know if the mood centers of my brain had been damaged, but I could definitely relate to several of those other possible causes. Plus, there was the heavy-duty pain medication I had been taking that probably contributed to the problem.

Just reading about TBIs and depression and the millions of people affected by them made me feel like I was in danger of having the sort of panic attack I'd had at the pain-management clinic. It was so distressing to know that the threat of depression was another lifelong issue I would have to deal with. In addition, I felt such empathetic sadness for all the other people who were suffering in the same way I was. So many millions of people were affected by TBI and depression, it seemed like a silent epidemic. If it was so widespread, why didn't people talk about it the way they did heart disease and cancer?

To pull myself out of my anxious state, I decided to pay attention to my breathing. I sucked air deep into my lungs and watched my stomach rise and fall with each breath. Even though I was able to avoid the panic attack, my life in general had become a deep blue and stormy ocean, where on good days I lay on the bottom and on bad days I burrowed beneath the sea floor.

I tried to climb back out of the blues but couldn't do it. I was willing myself to the store each day at this point, using every fiber of my being to put myself physically there, though my mind was elsewhere.

It was a particularly bleak day of sadness and side effects when two men pushed two other men in wheelchairs through the front door of Planet Futon. They parked the chairs near the front row of mattresses close to the window and proceeded to look around at the furniture, ignoring their charges. I greeted them all and gave the caregivers the rundown on our inventory. I didn't like that they were ignoring their patients, so I decided to walk over to them.

I approached the wheelchairs. One man was indifferent and uttered a small grunt as I said hello, but the other began making a lot of noise. He couldn't speak but it was clear he wanted to have some sort of interaction. In fact, vocally, he was really animated — and though none of the sounds could be understood as words, I just knew he wanted to have a conversation in some way. His eyes were lit up and he smiled through them, though his mouth was limp.

"You remind me of Dr. Stephen Hawking," I said to the man with the smiling eyes. It was not just because he was confined to a wheelchair; he really resembled him. "Do you like him?" He let out a stream of even greater enthusiastic sounds, which seemed to indicate that he did.

"Hi, I'm Jason." I continued, "You know, Dr. Hawking may be confined to a chair as well, but he speaks with his eyes, like you do. You can just see the intelligence behind them, like yours. I remember reading that he says his body may be trapped but his mind is free."

The man's eyes got wild with enthusiasm and he moaned loudly. His blue eyes finally stopped darting around and he stared deeply into mine. "I bet you have a lot of time to think," I said. "I've had a lot of time to think in my life too. I hardly left my house for nearly four years after a traumatic brain injury I suffered in a mugging. I would just sit and think and read and watch documentaries. Do you do a lot of thinking? I bet you know so many things with all that time to ponder." His eyes were moving again. Without him speaking, I knew when he meant yes and I knew when he didn't. This meant yes.

Then I could hardly believe it but he stared past me at the drawings on the wall behind the register and let out a deep groan.

"Are you looking at the drawings?"

Groan.

"I did them. I see these images in my mind synesthetically for numbers and equations. That one there is pi . . ."

With that, if the man could have leaped from his chair he would have, because he let out the loudest howl.

"Oh, you like pi?"

He howled again.

I launched into my usual enthusiastic explanation about the irrational number, but this time, I was careful not to sound too patronizing. I didn't want to talk down to this man. I felt the very cosmos behind those eyes of his.

When I finished, I told him I wished I could now listen to him teach me what he knew about pi. He let out the saddest little whimper.

The caregivers came over and told me that both clients suffered from cerebral palsy and that they lived in a facility nearby and were out for their daily walk.

The men then went back to looking at the furniture and I continued to discuss space-time, the Planck length, and relativity with the patient. The man's eyes stayed animated and enthusiastic for all of it. They practically sparkled.

The caregivers came over to take them back to their facility and thanked me for spending time with them. They pushed the men toward the door, and the one I'd had the conversation with kept me in his peripheral vision for as long as possible (he couldn't move his head). And then they were gone.

I walked into the storage room in back of the showroom because I didn't want any customers entering the store to see me crying. I was crying because I felt for the man in the wheelchair. I was crying at the memory of what his eyes looked like when I told him I'd also had a lot of time to think. And I was crying because I realized how lucky I was to be able-bodied. What torture it must be for him some days. What did I have to be upset about?

Jason, I said to myself, *snap out of it and stop complaining about things. Get to work!*

And with that, I pushed the mental and physical pain I was feeling aside, and as soon as all the customers left, I began again drafting what I would say about my experiences when I went to Stockholm.

CHAPTER FIFTEEN

Scandinavian Spring

I ENTERED THE LOBBY of the Kungsbron Hotel that chilly Scandinavian April like a dervish. I checked in, then immediately engaged anyone wearing a conference nametag in conversation, talking about my ideas and displaying my binder full of drawings. The place was buzzing — there were lots of people hanging out in clusters of animated discussion.

Maureen greeted me enthusiastically and immediately introduced me to Stuart Hameroff, the director of the conference, and Nick Day. Nick was a filmmaker specializing in the topic of consciousness and the director of the award-winning documentary *Short Cut to Nirvana: Kumbh Mela*. Dr. Hameroff was a professor of anesthesiology and psychology and the director for the Center for Consciousness Studies at the University of Arizona. Together they were collaborating on a full-length feature film called *Mindville,* about the mysteries of consciousness. They both greeted me warmly. Dr. Hameroff was soon pulled away by one of the dozens of other participants who wanted a word with him, which left me with Nick. I set my drawings out on a coffee table near the front desk and started from the beginning; three hours into my presentation to the patient Nick, I was still going strong. Nick invited me to be part of his documentary on the conference and wanted to do a special interview with me in *Consciousness Chronicles*, a series of films he'd been making for years that featured the speakers at these conferences. Just like that. Things moved fast from the beginning. You could feel the intellectual curiosity in the air, and there was a sense that people wanted to make the most of their week there. As I sat telling my story and explaining my drawings, I caught a glimpse of Deepak Chopra, and neuropsychiatrist Peter Fenwick walked by.

I also could not help but notice the frenetic pacing of a gray-haired man wearing a backward baseball cap nearby in the lobby.

His curls stuck out under the sides of his hat in Einstein-like poofs — if Einstein had co-opted the look started by professional baseball catchers, that is. You could tell he was deep in thought and should not be bothered at that moment. I learned this was physicist Allan Snyder, director of the Centre for the Mind at the University of Sydney, Australia. He was also cofounder of Emotiv Systems and winner of the 2001 Marconi Prize for his work in optical physics.

Dr. Snyder had been doing cutting-edge research on savant syndrome for more than a decade and suggested that savant skills were latent in everyone. Like several other scientists, he believed that the human brain typically filtered out many of the signals it received and focused on the information most necessary for survival. In his view, it was a failure of the brain to filter out that raw data that allowed savants to tap into the extraordinary innate skills within us all. But Dr. Snyder wasn't interested in the brains of savants alone. In fact, he had actually been trying to artificially induce savantism in normal people.

To do so, Dr. Snyder invented a creativity cap, which was intended to prod the brain to perform at savantlike levels. The device used a technique called transcranial direct-current stimulation that sent mild electrical jolts into the brain to alter activity within specific regions. Earlier models of the cap relied on magnetic stimulation to produce these results. In his experiments, people actually did better on tests while wearing the device and worse after they took it off. In one of Dr. Snyder's experiments that was particularly relevant to my case, he and his colleagues used his genius machine on a group of eleven people to see if it could improve their drawing skills. He fitted each nonsavant with the cap and then had him or her draw figures such as a dog, a horse, and a face. He tested each subject before, during, immediately following, and then forty-five minutes after using the device. The results? Immediately after the stimulator was applied, some of the participants displayed a higher level of drawing skills. The boost in ability disappeared forty-five minutes after the device was removed.

Dr. Snyder later said to Maureen that my case beautifully supported his hypothesis that it was possible to turn savant skills on and off in normal people. When I heard that, I wondered for a second if he knew a way to turn off my exhausting impressions, and I fantasized about asking him to do so, but then I decided I was happier the way I was.

I was soon joined by Paul Synowiec, the videographer I'd hired to track me at the conference. To save money, he and I would be sharing a room—something that would be very difficult for me, given my phobia of other people's germs. I could not have asked for a better roommate, though. From the start, Paul was very sensitive to my OCD and checked in frequently to make sure I was doing okay. He put me most at ease by actually swabbing things down with rubbing alcohol; he sterilized everything from the faucet handles to the doorknobs. I couldn't believe he'd thought of that. He was extra-clean and worked hard to stay on his side of the room so I wouldn't be nervous.

After talking with Nick that first night, I realized the other synesthetes had already found one another and were among the most intimate of the groups. Some of them knew one another already from other conferences and from lively online communities dedicated to their abilities. I began to bond with some of them in the hotel lobby and in nearby restaurants and taverns, where we all spent every moment of free time. I hadn't realized that so many people were actually very comfortable with their synesthesia; people who were born with a version of what I was experiencing seemed much more at home in their skin than I felt sometimes, as this was still very new to me. By getting to know them, I was reminded that synesthesia can take dozens of forms. They were excited when they did presentations on their abilities, but in private, they were more blasé about them than I was. Still, I was not strange to this band of brothers and sisters who spoke offhandedly among themselves about the photisms they saw—the shapes and the colors that existed out in space or in their minds' eyes. They welcomed me warmly and immediately. Even though my case was "extraordinary," it was not so hard to explain things to them because of our shared impressions. Though not all synesthetes are savants—most are believed to be average to above average in intelligence—I found them exceptional. Most of them took very readily to my ideas. Perhaps this was because I'd rendered my concepts in drawings, and synesthetes are known to be gifted in the arts.

I finally met the distinguished scientist and synesthete Dr. Neil Theise, who had earlier so graciously spent time talking to me about his theories and findings on meditation, synesthesia, consciousness, and the mind. I'd really been looking forward to meeting him in person. He nodded when I explained the shapes I saw out in space around me. Dr. Theise, who was a pioneer in the field of adult stem-cell plasticity, said he saw shapes too; his days and weeks and months extended around him like wheels. He was like a hamster inside a wheel. When he wanted to go to a particular time on a particular day, he simply flicked his spatial wheel and locked in on the exact unit he wanted.

Dr. Theise and I shared a hero in Einstein. In one of his thought experiments, Einstein had famously imagined riding on a light beam, and he'd had some of his inspirations about special relativity in that vision. Similarly, Dr. Theise said that he'd imagined himself riding a stem cell, and he'd had inspirations about their plasticity in that state.

During the conference, I met so many amazing people. It was as if I was making up for all those years I'd spent in isolation. There was German synesthete Alexandra Kirschner, a sweet pixie of a singing instructor for a boys' choir near Stuttgart. She explained to me that she identified child synesthetes in her chorus and taught them to sing by telling them to go to the green, round note or the pink, triangular one instead of saying middle C. She planned to sing as part of her presentation and I was told this would be exceptional, given the perfect acoustics of Aula Magna, Stockholm University's auditorium, combined with Alexandra's considerable talent. She was very funny. She gave a running commentary on what was going on by making shadow puppets of her hands and changing her voice for each character; her right hand was a fictional German newscaster she'd created, Paul Nachricht, and her left was his opinionated and tress-obsessed wife, Olga. "Synesthesia Gang going to lunch now," reported Paul. "It's snowing. What about my hair?" responded Olga, knowing she'd have to come along, affixed to the end of Alexandra's wrist as she was.

As comical as this fräulein could be, I learned she had a very sensitive, philosophical side as well. For example, she noted that the visual imagery of young synesthetes in her care was richer than that of adults — perhaps owing to childhood imagination. She would love for researchers to look into this further and develop teaching models around it. Alexandra didn't learn that what she had was called synesthesia until 2006, when she read an article in which a person described a 5 as yellow. She herself saw 5 as red. She also had colored letters, weekdays, months, music, sounds, and smells. She called me tenderhearted and said that I stood out even among the wonderful, open members of the U.S. delegation of synesthetes at the conference. I was touched when she told me she was moved by both the complexity of my mathematics and the way I described my mugging and injury. "Together, we are all like different musical instruments in the same orchestra to my mind," she exclaimed. "Jason, you are the trumpet!"

The American artist and synesthete Carrie C. Firman was well known and respected in the community for her work, so I was really happy to meet her. One outstanding piece, titled "Sympathy Pains," she'd created was a trench coat she fitted with LED lights that glowed in the colors she actually saw around her body in response to pain. Carrie, who made some of the most beautiful and realistic renderings of what synesthetic photisms look like in her photographic series *That Which Cannot Be Said with Words* (which was displayed in the conference's art gallery), suffered chronic pain from an illness and for every hurt she felt on her body, she saw a color out in the space around her. She made a jacket fitted with bags of rice to indicate the discomfort and awkwardness of her own painful movements and wore the jacket when she exhibited her art sometimes, but unfortunately she didn't bring it to Stockholm, so I've only seen pictures of her wearing it. I really admired and related to Carrie. We both had had to work through chronic pain. And we both worked diligently to record what we see through art.

Israeli synesthete and psychotherapist Naama Kostiner and I began to develop a meaningful friendship early on. She talked about integrating holistic techniques, including color therapy, into modern-day psychotherapy. I found her very bright and open.

I shared some highlights of my life story with her behind the scenes and she provided wonderful insights.

Whenever we spoke, I became more relaxed. After noticing my difficulty sitting outside on public benches or riding the metro back to the hotel, she asked if I would be more comfortable sitting outside in nature.

"Sure, if it's a green meadow or under a nice tree, where people don't tend to pass and contaminate the place, I'd love to." I also told her that I had no problem touching my wife, Elena, someone I love and trust completely.

When I said this, a look of realization dawned on her face. After thinking for a moment, Naama said, "Jason, I think your greatest fear is of people and not of open spaces or germs. The night of the mugging, you were intentionally hurt by people and then your friends didn't help. Of course this made you question people's moral character and compassion, and you developed a distrust of humankind. This explains your willingness to explore 'untouched' or 'undamaged' nature and be intimate with your wife, the one person you truly trust in the world. Washing your hands seems like a ritual, cleansing yourself from 'evil, contaminated' society."

I told Naama that I thought there might be truth to her theory. I later demonstrated my trust in her by giving her a hug.

It was good to finally meet Dr. Brogaard, or Brit, as she asked me to call her, with whom I would co-present in a Q-and-A format at Aula Magna and in a workshop prior to that. We would then travel on to Helsinki. The Copenhagen-born researcher was quite at home in Scandinavia and had lots of experience presenting at other conferences. We practiced our presentation many times before the big moment — having Brit ask me questions to prompt portions of my story helped us fit everything into the twenty-minute time slot, as I'm prone to go on and on about the things I'm passionate about.

That evening, our rainbow tribe walked off together, several members chattering on about their respective colors for numbers and letters, their shapes for time, and how they feel music. Alexandra, the singing instructor, saw the look of wonder and excitement on my face, whipped out her shadow-puppet hand, and, in an attempt at a police dispatcher's voice, said, "Spotted walking south in Stockholm: the Synesthesia Gang. Armed with many shapes in the air around them. Approach cautiously. *Very dangerous!*" I laughed a deep belly laugh and the private joke persisted long after Stockholm. There are even Synesthesia Gang T-shirts now. She later told Maureen she liked me a lot and loved my silvery-gray voice in particular.

Over dinner, my new friends talked about Dr. Cytowic, the neurology professor and pioneer in modern synesthesia research I had read about when I first started learning about this. The group was so reverent, they spoke almost in whispers when they talked about him. He believed that synesthesia might be going on in all of us, but only a small percentage got a conscious bleed that resulted in the kind of imagery seen by synesthetes.

In a 1995 paper for the journal *Psyche,* Dr. Cytowic explained this idea by comparing synesthetic perception to a TV transmission. What we see on the TV screen is the end result of a broadcast, and most people are able to see only this final product. But what if someone could intercept the broadcast before it ever reached the TV screen? The transmission might be in a different, perhaps more raw form. He suggested that this might be how synesthetes view things. This made me think of those images I've seen of a television director looking at dozens of monitors and choosing which feeds will end up on a news broadcast. Maybe synesthetes are like those directors, seeing more than one feed at a time.

I also learned over dinner how synesthetic images often act as mnemonic devices. The group discussed Solomon Veniaminovich Shereshevsky, a Russian journalist who became known as a memory whiz. For decades, Russian neuropsychologist and memory researcher Alexander Luria studied the young man, eventually writing a book about him, published in English in 1968, called *The Mind of a Mnemonist: A Little Book about a Vast Memory*. At one point,

Dr. Luria claimed that S., as he referred to his subject, "probably possesses the strongest memory of all men." For example, he could look at extensive lists of numbers for mere moments and then repeat them all — even in reverse — and he could memorize lengthy passages of famous literary works in foreign languages even though he didn't speak those languages.

In his efforts to determine how Shereshevsky was able to perform such incredible feats of memory, Luria discovered that he had a sort of all-encompassing synesthesia involving all five senses. The stimulation of one sense might cause reactions in a number of the others. For example, if he heard a musical note, he might see a color, feel a touch, or taste something. He also personified numbers — the number 1 was a proud, well-built man; the number 2 was a high-spirited woman; and so on — which helped him remember series of numbers quite readily. I could relate to that. I had found that I could remember phone numbers much more easily now — it must have to do with the associated shapes for the numbers, which underscore them somehow.

The group talked about how these extrasensory responses acted as mnemonics for all of us as they did for Shereshevsky. We spent a while discussing things that had become indelible in our minds because of the extra associations. Maureen told the story of how in grade school, she was stuck on a test question about when the United States had entered World War I. "I couldn't remember the year, but I knew it was ebony-umber-ebony-scarlet, so I worked backwards to 1914."

I contributed that my hero Daniel Tammet, the synesthete and savant, wrote in his memoir *Born on a Blue Day* that he saw numbers not only as shapes and colors but also as textures and motions. Even more interesting was the fact that for him, numbers had their own personalities — some were loud (5), some were shy (4), some were small (6), some were big (23), some were ugly (289), and some were beautiful (333). Considering that this was how Tammet perceived numbers, it's not surprising that he had an emotional response to them. My favorite thing about Tammet, though, was that, like me, he was fascinated by the number pi, so much so that he devoted an entire chapter of his memoir to it. I am in awe of the fact that in March 2004, he recited pi from memory and got to 22,514 digits in just five hours and nine minutes—a European record!

We walked back to the hotel, and though I was intent on having a restful night, I found myself overstimulated and worried about the fact that I was sharing the space with a roommate. I slathered antibacterial lotion over my whole body before putting on my pajamas and lying down for a fitful night, despite the heroic efforts of my bunkmate, Paul.

The next day arrived too soon, although I couldn't help but find the nerves exhilarating. It reminded me of when I'd taken the stage as Oliver or jumped out of planes. Paul and I went to Aula Magna and walked onstage to get a sense of it before the actual presentation. He even did a handstand when no one was looking so that he could say he did. Laughing at that released a lot of tension for me.

As I was about to walk out onto the stage for my debut, a spotlight shone in my eyes, and its rays fanned out over the wooden relief work of the theater in a perfect, demarcated polygon. I whispered, "Look, Maureen, it's pi." She looked up, nodded, and broke into a wide smile. "Good luck, Jason," she whispered back. "You can do this!"

Finally in front of an audience of academics, with no futons to ring up at the end of the conversation, I was about to launch my career as a theorist. People fumbled with papers and talked a little, and then I began. I opened with the story of my mugging a decade ago. The audience grew silent. I noticed a number of them nodding at me, offering encouragement. The rest of the panel members on the stage were also nodding. I *can* do this!

The PowerPoint then opened to my drawings as I explained everything from pi onward, guided by Brit's questions. People started to wander into the talk — some just stood in the doorways and aisles. I felt like I'd crossed a huge finish line when people applauded at the end and I made my way back to my seat. Life would be different from now on, of that I was sure.

I got terrific feedback about my participation at the conference and discovered that many people were talking about me. Nick Day, the filmmaker I spoke to at length the first night of the conference, said, "Jason's case is extremely rare, if not unique ... If our world presents a smooth and contiguous surface, Jason's reveals the deeper substructure of geometric forms and patterns, of pixels and grids and lattices ..."

Nick also talked about how I fit into the ongoing exploration of consciousness — whether it is merely a byproduct of brain activity, as most traditional scientists believe, or whether it is more fundamental than that, as some esoteric theorists suggest. He thought that either theory could explain my situation. I was honored to think that a few of these amazing scientists might actually look to me as some sort of living proof of their complex theories about the most essential questions about the mind.

Even the conference director, Dr. Hameroff, had something to say about me after the meeting: "Synesthetic minds plumb deeper order, finer scales of consciousness. Jason Padgett's savant synesthesia suggests the mind, reality and the universe are fractal-like, and self-similar." Yes! Hearing this from such an important person reinforced my belief that the visions I was seeing were perhaps the very fabric of the universe.

I was both exhilarated by my debut in Stockholm and nervous about what would be next. What would the tests in Helsinki show about my mind? There was no turning back from the truth now.

CHAPTER SIXTEEN

Traveling Without Moving

LEFT STOCKHOLM ON May 8 and boarded a plane for another Scandinavian hub of consciousness: Helsinki, Finland. Brit, who had been my co-presenter at the conference, arranged with a team of neuroscientists to put me through my paces at Aalto University. While we could have done the tests in America, Brit had an association with the Scandinavian lab, and it was expedient to do it while we were all together in Europe. The tall, blond Danish philosopher and scientist and I were so engaged in conversation on the plane that we walked right through customs without our luggage and had to circle back.

I was nervous about being in a new place. Some posttraumatic stress struck as I was out and about in Helsinki, and I felt afraid of strangers. I was also prickly about taking the tests and discovering the truth, which would be revealed through brain scans done by high-tech machines. Would it confirm what I suspected? Or would the scientists see something terribly wrong when they finally got a glimpse of my gray matter?

Brit took the time to explain how important it was for others to understand what I experienced. "No one knows exactly how people with savant syndrome are able to do the amazing things they do," she wrote to me and Maureen. "But everyone agrees that we won't have a good picture of how the human brain functions until we know how they do it."

One of Brit's hypotheses was that people with savant syndrome had conscious access to parts of the brain that normal people didn't. She explained that the brain did many calculations throughout the day — think of something as simple as reaching for a computer mouse and moving it around. While we can feel our movements, most people don't have access to the inner calculations their brains are performing to make the movement possible. She said that these calculations take place in the dorsal stream, also referred to as the where/how pathway, which runs from the visual cortex at the back of the head upward through the parietal cortex near the top of the head. Most people have access to the output only, not the calculations. "But people with savant syndrome of a mathematical kind apparently are able to use these areas of the brain to calculate amazing things," she explained. She hypothesized that savants gained conscious access to the process through synesthetic visualizations. The "zombie calculations" that take place in hidden areas of the brain are translated into pictures, colors, and shapes, she said. This made a lot of sense to me, since I saw pictures for my math constantly. "Synesthesia is a kind of gateway into the hidden areas of our brains," she said.

I was starting to really appreciate the combination of things I'd acquired. I might not have become a savant without the synesthetic imagery that allowed me to show my process and create my art. I was grateful I had both now, despite the tradeoffs.

Even though I had just arrived in Helsinki, the testing process had actually begun several months earlier. Prior to my trip, as part of my evaluation for synesthesia, I was asked to draw a wheel, a balloon, and my interpretation of a mathematical formula. Approximately three months later, I was asked to draw the same things. The drawings would be compared for consistency as part of the testing process, which also included the brain-imaging scans I was about to undergo.

When we entered the lab, it was humming with human activity and machinery. I told the researchers that I liked to think I was smart now, but the people who created such diagnostics and used them were the true geniuses.

They told me that the whole wing of the center was shielded with metal in order to keep radio-frequency waves from interfering with the equipment's readings. I would be tested with both functional magnetic resonance imaging, which would provide a general view of the activity in my brain, and transcranial magnetic stimulation (TMS), which would isolate what was going on in specific areas in greater detail.

First up was the fMRI. What makes fMRI such a useful tool is that it reveals images of the brain in action. In everyday life, when you do ordinary things — calculate a 15 percent tip at a restaurant, figure out an alternative route home when there's a traffic jam, or have a conversation — specific areas of the brain are activated. To help neurons do their job, oxygen-rich blood flow increases in those areas. Using radio waves and a powerful magnetic field, fMRI measures and maps brain activity by detecting these changes in blood flow. Active areas of the brain appear to light up on the three-dimensional scans produced by the high-tech machines, providing a glimpse of how the brain functions.

I put on a white jumpsuit that made me feel like an astronaut. It was the longest journey I would ever take without moving — a voyage to the truth. First, the scientists scanned me with the fMRI. I was not terribly claustrophobic in the enclosed space; it felt similar to the MRI I'd undergone years ago. It took about forty minutes, but I was so deep in thought, the time seemed to fly by in just a few minutes. When I was in the machine, the researchers flashed many images onto a screen in front of my eyes, including objects like leaves, seashells, a screw, human faces showing varying emotions, a rubber duckie, numbers, and formulas. There was even an image of a grenade! While most people would associate the last item with war and destruction, I found myself transfixed by the fractal nature of the designs on its outer shell. I wondered what the researchers were seeing in my brain while I was pondering the images. I couldn't feel anything going on, but things were lighting up on the monitors outside my view. I heard a humming sound even through my earplugs and saw waves go by in my mind's eye that must have been a synesthetic reaction of some sort.

The next day I had a second fMRI, and the day after that, I had the TMS test. TMS is a noninvasive way to change how neurons act in the brain. It delivers quick magnetic pulses to targeted areas of brain tissue to stimulate the nerve cells. A form of TMS called repetitive TMS (rTMS) is sometimes used as a treatment for depression and other neurological and psychiatric disorders. It is also one of the techniques Dr. Snyder, the curly-haired man I saw at the conference who is the director of the Centre for the Mind in Australia, used in his attempts to induce savantlike skills in nonsavants. In my case, it would be used to inhibit regions identified in the fMRI so the researchers could see if that would diminish the synesthesia.

For this test, I was told I wouldn't need to lie down in a machine. Instead, the TMS device, which looked like a paddle with two loops, would be placed near my head as I sat in a chair. Short bursts of current would be used to inhibit my brain's activity in specific areas so the scientists could find the neural correlates of synesthesia induced by mathematical formulas they showed me.

One of the neuroscientists fitted me with the world's funkiest glasses — oversize, gray, and angular — before putting the paddle device and its inner coils near, but not touching, my head. The glasses would flash the images to stimulate my brain.

"You look like Anakin Skywalker!" he said.

"Now, *this* is pod-racing," I joked, alluding to the sport loved by the George Lucas hero; the races had always thrilled me as a moviegoer, but they paled in comparison to this. When the neuroscientist told me he'd never actually seen a Star Wars film, I clutched my chest like I was having a heart attack. I am a devoted fan of the series.

I had read that the TMS would be only minimally uncomfortable, but I noticed I got zapped lightly by the device. It reminded me of the time my troublesome brother hit me with a stun gun; thankfully, this was much less intense.

When it was all finally over, I couldn't wait to see what the tests would reveal. To be able to grasp the information, though, I first had to understand a few basics about the brain, such as the concepts of left brain and right brain. Neuroscientists have long believed that the left hemisphere of the brain is involved in processes that are analytical, logical, and detail-oriented, while the right hemisphere tends to see the big picture, recognize patterns, and contribute to creativity. Newer research on the differences between the left brain and right brain have shown that the distinctions may not be as clear-cut as once thought. And of course, both sides of the brain communicate with each other, thanks in large part to the corpus callosum, a thick band of more than two hundred million nerve fibers that connect the two hemispheres.

This left brain/right brain stuff was important because many studies on savants have shown damage in the left hemisphere of the brain. There are a number of theories about what this means and what role it plays in acquired savantism or acquired synesthesia. Would one of these theories be the answer to the mystery of my brain?

Some scientists claim that the left side of the brain typically inhibits, or suppresses, activity on the right side. As Brit explained it, "The left hemisphere normally keeps the right hemisphere under

control, but when there is a lesion or a disturbance in the left hemisphere, suddenly the right hemisphere is 'out of the tyranny' of the
left and can develop hidden abilities." Is that what happened to me?
Had my left brain relinquished control of my right brain?

Other experts, such as Dr. Snyder, suggest that it's the left hemisphere that filters out much of the raw sensory data the brain de-
tects. So when there are problems on the left side of the brain, the
filter can go on the fritz. In a 2009 paper that appeared in *Philosophical Transactions of the Royal Society*, Snyder claimed it was
this failure that allowed for conscious awareness of the unfiltered
material. This is in line with what Dr. Bushell said, that the human retina is capable of seeing things at the quantum level but that
the brain filters out what is considered unnecessary. Had my filters
been damaged, allowing the raw material to flood in?

Brit thought there was another mechanism at work. As she had
already explained to me, she believed synesthesia played a role in
some people gaining access to the inner zombie calculations that
most others aren't aware of. But that's not all. In an interview with
Popular Science, she explained, "When brain cells die, they release
a barrage of neurotransmitters, and this deluge of potent chemicals
may actually rewire parts of the brain, opening up new neural path-
ways into areas previously unavailable." Had neurotransmitters in
the injured areas of my brain spilled into other regions of my brain
and caused some changes there?

Research from Dr. Treffert indicated that when some areas of
the brain were damaged, other areas were recruited to compensate, which may give rise to savant abilities. However, in an article
he wrote, called "The Savant Syndrome," he noted that "no single
theory can explain all savants." Did this mean that more than one
theory could apply to me? Or that something completely different
might have occurred in my case?

I was about to find out.

When my results were in, I felt so excited. After waiting nearly ten long years, I was finally going to discover what had happened to my brain. I noticed that Brit was excited too. She said she had been waiting her whole life for a case like mine and that the results were amazing.

As I looked at my brain scans, I saw splashes of yellow, orange, and red. These were the active areas that had lit up in response to the mathematical formulas they showed me in the fMRI. I couldn't wait for Brit to tell me what it all meant.

She explained it to me and later summed it all up in an e-mail to Maureen. She even published an article in the journal *Neurocase* about her findings.

She started out by saying that when my brain was being scanned to detect the neurological underpinnings of my synesthesia, there was activation in some of the areas of the temporal lobes, frontal lobes, and parietal cortex, an area that most people don't have conscious access to. She wrote, "The parietal lobe is where sensory information is integrated from various parts of the body, but more importantly in Jason's case, it's also where knowledge of numbers and their relations resides." She explained that in being able to consciously access math processes, I was actually seeing behind the curtain into how math works. The areas of the parietal cortex were activated when I was looking at mathematical formulas that gave rise to fractal imagery but not when I was shown nonsense formulas.

Hearing this news, I felt like Dorothy looking behind the curtain at the Wizard of Oz — except I was not disappointed with what I saw. What a privilege to be able to not only do math but see it at every step and even draw its geometric foundations.

"Even more surprising is that when Jason was looking at the stimuli which give rise to fractal images in him, he used only his left hemisphere to generate the synesthesia," Brit continued. "When he was looking at nonsense formulas, he used both hemispheres."

This was the reverse of what the neuroscientists expected. Ordinarily, as previous brain-imaging studies had shown, the right hemisphere is dominant in people with savant syndrome; that's most likely due to damage to the left side. Once again, I didn't fit the mold. Brit explained what this might mean for me.

"Exact mathematics is much more of a left-hemisphere activity whereas approximate mathematics (how many birds on a wire, how many apples in a bowl) happens in both hemispheres," Brit wrote. "Jason is more engaged by exact math in the left hemisphere."

Apparently I had received more damage to the right side of my brain, specifically to areas of the visual cortex, which is involved in detecting motion and boundaries. Because of this, there was a possibility my left side was compensating, Brit explained. She also noted that the hyperactive areas of my brain are located next to those that were injured. This is important because it fits in with her hypothesis that dying brain cells release a flood of neurotransmitters into neighboring regions that may ultimately rewire the brain. In my case, the areas that became highly active were probably right in the path of the rush of neurotransmitters.

Finally, after all these years, I had an official diagnosis. Based on my brain scans as well as those drawings I had done months earlier, Brit found that I had conceptual, or higher, synesthesia, as opposed to the more common perceptual, or lower, form. And to the best of her knowledge, I was the first person who had ever acquired both synesthesia and savant syndrome. More than that, I was apparently the first to hand-draw mathematical fractals and the first known synesthete to see objects and formulas as fractals.

I was so happy to know that what I was experiencing was legitimate, wasn't mental illness, and was, in fact, extraordinary. It felt wonderful to be "proven." I'd never had the evidence beyond my own behavior and experiences until then. It was real; it had been proven scientifically! I'd always felt in the core of my being something like this was going on, but due to some of the reactions of others — including that nameless professor who told me there was something wrong with my brain — I'd also always had a bit of doubt. I left Helsinki for home more confident in my abilities and motivated to use my acquired savant syndrome and synesthesia for good.

CHAPTER SEVENTEEN

Pilgrimage to Wisconsin

NOW FELT LIKE I had proof of my unlikely gifts. It was hard to return to my life managing the futon business. My Scandinavian journey proved to me that I had to carve out a new path in life, but I had many responsibilities I couldn't walk away from. I now truly wanted to change my profession to something more suitable for my new interests and abilities. I also thought I needed to change my living environment. I knew there were more inspiring places Elena and I could live.

Maureen had interviewed the savant Daniel Tammet for her first book and pointed out that he, too, ultimately left a hardscrabble working-class environment in London for greener pastures more suitable to his sensitivities. He now lives in the heart of Paris.

He told her he felt stunted as a child due to his autism. He wasn't very open to the world in his youth, not even the world of art. "I was very much in retreat," he said. "But since then the evolution has been a result of a lot of work, a lot of love, and a lot of effort, and today, art plays a big role in my life — all kinds of art: painting, literature, and so on."

Like Daniel, I needed to find my higher ground. I found a really good salesman whom I believed I could train to take over for me in the futon stores one day as manager, and that was a huge step in the right direction. He and I began looking for some great salespeople to add to the staff. However, I was still having some health issues and trying to stop taking prescription pain medicines. Between work and health problems, I couldn't return to school yet. There were two groups of sufferers I could relate to now: people with TBIs, and people with chronic pain who got hooked on prescription medication. These two things clamped down on my life like a giant vise.

I wanted to continue moving toward becoming the new me, however. One thing I wanted to do to put a final stamp of approval on my acquired conditions and give me more insight was visit the man who had offered me so much hope in my years of isolation: psychiatrist Darold Treffert, the world authority on savants. I'd found Dr. Treffert to be a paternal and caring physician during our previous phone conversations. If there was one person who could point the way forward, it was this octogenarian in Wisconsin. I'm not being facetious or religious when I say that receiving a confirmation of my diagnosis from him would be akin to getting the pope's blessing. I wanted to see him partly because he was an internationally renowned medical professional but also because I had the feeling that this was where it had all started for me — seeing him on the television program with Tammet had been my first hint that I might be a synesthete and a savant.

Maureen made the arrangements around Dr. Treffert's busy schedule in late October 2012 and we agreed to fly from our respective coasts and meet in Chicago. From there, we would drive the rest of the way together to Fond du Lac, a beautiful little town whose name means "Foot of the Lake" that's situated on the southern shore of Lake Winnebago.

We were not there long when I declared, "I could totally live here!" It is a picturesque and friendly place, and I fell in love with it.

We planned to meet the doctor at a restaurant he'd recommended called Theo's. I found myself a little nervous to finally greet him face-to-face. He'd examined and befriended so many extraordinary savants in his career, some four hundred in fifty years. Only thirty of them had acquired savantism later in life. He'd written authoritative books on the topic, including *Islands of Genius* and *Extraordinary People*, as well as countless academic papers. How would I measure up?

In *Islands of Genius*, Dr. Treffert called people like me halfway savants — the *halfway* not an indicator of abilities but a reference to having fewer tradeoffs than those born with savant syndrome. Even though I now suffer from OCD, PTSD, and extreme empathy, among other things, I do think I've had only minor cognitive and neuropsychological reactions to my injuries compared to other savants.

Maureen and I walked into Theo's, and there at the bar nursing an ice water was the unmistakable white-haired man, as big as a bear and with a kindly smile. We said hello and he stood and I felt he was as large as his renown; he simply towered over us. After a warm handshake from him, I felt all of my nervousness dissipate.

We were seated for dinner and were joined by a colleague from Stockholm, Carrie C. Firman, the synesthetic artist; she was now teaching in nearby Madison.

It was a fascinating night: Dr. Treffert spoke on the many cases he'd had over the decades and took the time to ask about the types of synesthesia of all present. We finished up early, our bellies full of Wisconsin cheese-connoisseur favorites like Parmesan fries and beer-cheese soup. We planned to meet him at his office at St. Agnes

Hospital the next morning at 9:00 for my formal interview. Then we'd have lunch at a church-turned-restaurant called Trinity and go on to his home office for further discussion.

I was tingling when I rose the next morning, and it was not the muscle tremors but the anticipation I felt about finally sitting down officially with the dean of savants. Maureen and I made our way over to the hospital, and Dr. Treffert greeted us in the glass-enclosed, light-filled modern lobby. First he walked us into a chapel to show us the labyrinth on the floor that people use for meditation there. He pointed out how much it looked like my drawings. He was right. I had never seen a more meaningful or intriguing space; it even had a waterfall that pulled my eye as much as the geometry of the labyrinth, given how much I love to watch flowing water. We headed to the hospital library and took our seats at a round wooden table.

We began the conversation with my talking about the night of the mugging. It all came back into scary focus as I described the sights and smells and sounds. I answered questions about my complicated family history, my previous and current interests, and my new abilities. After having me demonstrate some of my drawing ability about an hour into our meeting, Dr. Treffert paused to reflect:

"I think your case is truly amazing: the suddenness of it; the drama of your drawings as well as your newfound arithmetic ability is in itself startling. And there is also very little tradeoff of other abilities, which I think is encouraging . . . In that sense I think you're a really good ambassador for traumatic brain injury individuals — showing a great deal of optimism and hope and indeed overcoming what happened."

Listening to him made me realize yet again that I was more fortunate than many. I was also encouraged to hear that although Dr. Treffert knew I had many tradeoffs, he considered them relatively minimal.

After lunch, we followed Dr. Treffert's SUV, with its SAVANTS license plate, out to his home, which was set on several acres of prime woodland. When I was a kid, my dad had an RV and took my family to every state, and this part of the country was as pretty as any I'd ever seen. We passed patchwork fields of farms on the highway and soon arrived at his residence. In a clearing on one side of his house, he had an orchard filled with many varieties of fruit trees, and he took us on a walk on a trail just beyond his home, a wide, level path where a railroad track had once been. We hiked across a bridge, and ahead of us to the left was the most picturesque waterfall. Even at a late-fall trickle, it was breathtaking. I saw, within the outcroppings of the rocks there, the webby water features I began every morning with when I turned on the bathroom faucet. In this setting, they were even more tantalizing.

Dr. Treffert walked us back to his home and gave us signed copies of *Islands of Genius*. I was allergic to his cat so I waited downstairs near his office while Maureen toured the inside of the well-appointed home with him and his charming wife, Dorothy. I turned to the chapter in his book that had meant so much to me. His summary filled me with a sense of pride and wonder:

"Acquired" savant syndrome or "accidental genius" is the most important new development in the study of savant syndrome since it was first described over a century ago. It is particularly important to note how many such cases include *left* (dominant) *hemisphere dysfunction* with the release of dormant *right* (non-dominant) *hemisphere capacity* (paradoxical functional facilitation) as opposed to development of entirely new skills. In some instances there is a noticeable diminution of certain cognitive or other abilities with the emergence of new skills (acquired savant) but in other cases only minor, barely significant, detrimental trade-off occurs and these persons continue to function at a very high level overall ("halfway" savant).

Even though the brain testing I had undergone in Helsinki had shown that this description didn't exactly fit what had happened to my brain, the passage still made me realize how special and rare this all was.

We spent our last night in Wisconsin at the American Club in nearby Kohler, Wisconsin, a town named for the plumbing-and-housewares manufacturer headquartered there. Dr. Treffert should really be the governor of Wisconsin, or at least its tourism director, because he showed us so many of the highlights of his region. The American Club is a luxury spa and resort now but it was built in 1918 to house the poor immigrant workers employed by the company's founder. As we ascended the stairs at the club, I could almost hear their weary voices echoing through the remaining exposed brick that lent so much character to the place.

As we entered the dining room, however, I saw why it was the Midwest's only AAA Five Diamond resort hotel — it was brimming with custom woodwork, tapestries, and fine furniture.

Dr. Treffert ordered his standard drink, not an ice water this time but an old-fashioned, and Maureen and I got the same. We toasted our meeting, and I wasn't sure if it was the whiskey or the company, but I felt more warm and relaxed than I had in ages. Meeting Dr. Treffert and having his imprimatur on my case meant the world to me. I felt part of a rare fraternity now.

CHAPTER EIGHTEEN

No Regrets

AFTER YEARS OF speculation and confusion, I finally have a fledgling sense of a real identity. I feel optimistic, thanks to my conference debut, the new community of synesthetes around me, the findings of the first detailed scans of my brain, and especially my meeting with the legendary Dr. Treffert. It's like I've just been formally introduced to my new self after years of having two beings co-inhabit my battered body: the old me and the suddenly new me. I'm ready to remember the way I was without regret and move on more fully into the unexplored territory that is me *now*: the world's only known person with acquired savant syndrome and acquired synesthesia.

Based on everything I've learned so far, I have to agree with Dr. Treffert's and Dr. Snyder's theory that the visions I (and my fellow synesthetes) see and the capabilities I (and my fellow savants) have are available to everyone. I believe I am living proof that these powers lie dormant in all of us. Given my anemic educational background prior to my attack, nothing in my life up to that point could account for these abilities. Not a thing was added; rather, the knowledge was uncovered from some deep and mysterious place.

Just ask my parents. "You knew no mathematical terms at all before this; none, zero," my dad said when I asked him what he thought of the changes in me. "The math is a complete right turn — you're going down the highway and then just turn ninety degrees differently. It opened up an intellectual window that wasn't there before. It's pretty remarkable. I'm a pretty analytical guy so I wouldn't call it a miracle. But it's something."

My mom was just as surprised by my new abilities and interests. "It was like a fountain had been turned on flowing out of your mouth, your ears, your skin, with information coming faster than you could keep up with," she said. "You can't look at anything without seeing the underlying geometry of it. Maybe I need the tint you have on your glasses on mine!"

As for the scientists, they're still working on their theories to explain what happened in my brain. Dr. Treffert contends that genetic memory was released as my brain rewired itself and healed. As he wrote in his book *Islands of Genius*, "Genetic memory is simply the biological transfer of *knowledge, templates, and certain skills* along with the myriad of other inherited physical characteristics, instincts, traits, and behaviors." This genetic memory isn't a Padgett family heirloom being passed from one generation to the next in my family tree, but rather a shared genetic memory among all of humankind. It's as if we all come preloaded with this knowledge. The idea that human DNA might come with some sort of blueprint of hidden capabilities fascinates me most of all.

Dr. Treffert taught me about the three R's as they pertain to what happened to my brain. They stand for brain *rewiring, recruitment* of unused capacity, and *release* of dormant potential. Though these are present in people who are born with savant syndrome, he explained, their existence has been severely underestimated in the rest of us. Cases like mine prove a far greater plasticity of the brain in its ability to heal itself than was previously thought. He said that this has implications not only for brain-injury survivors like me but also for those who have autism, neurological damage from strokes, or nervous system disorders. This makes me feel hopeful that my experience may one day help other people.

I've learned so much on this journey. To be one person and then, suddenly, to become another has given me the ability to empathize with a wide range of people. Before my injury, I did not have much interest in, or patience for, those who pursued academic knowledge. Now I have the highest respect for such people. Similarly, I have empathy for young people who get a little lost in the party scene and lose their way academically. I may not be like them anymore, but I have thought about how that can deaden a lot of pain and keep one afloat during difficult times.

And where my communication with other people was once often superficial, if pleasant, I now have almost daily conversations with the customers at my store about the very meaning of life and how the universe works. My art is central to sharing these ideas with others. To me it is the fundamental nature of things, but will it end up shedding light on the nature of the cosmos when considered by top mathematicians and astrophysicists? I would like to start that conversation and humbly share whatever is going on in my mind with key people from many fields. To me, the beauty and symmetry of what I see and draw signals some greater truth. Dr. Jean-Pierre Luminet, the French astrophysicist, writer, and poet, considered geometric art's importance in his 2009 paper "Science, Art and Geometrical Imagination." He said, "Modern physicists such as John Wheeler and Roger Penrose insist on the significance of aesthetics in choosing and evaluating scientific theories. According to Penrose, 'It is a mysterious thing, in fact, how something which looks attractive may have a better chance of being true than something which looks ugly.'"

I agree with this assessment. To me, the truth of what I'm seeking lies in the beauty of what I see. In his new book *Measurement,* mathematician Paul Lockhart also supports this idea. "What makes a mathematician," he wrote, "is not technical skill or encyclopedic knowledge but insatiable curiosity and a desire for simple beauty."

I still have so much more to learn. I need more background in mathematics and physics and supporting subjects in order to better understand the value of what I'm seeing and drawing. My new wetware didn't come with an instruction manual, but I believe that more formal study of these subjects will allow me to wield my new talents with greater clarity and focus.

If nature really does reveal herself through exceptions, as the famous maxim says, what is nature trying to tell us through my example?

Here's what I think, from inside this rare thing: The way I see the world is visual proof to me that we are all enmeshed in a geometric space, and we are all capable of knowing more about it. I'm not talking about just studying theoretical models. I'm talking about witnessing them through personal experience. But to do so, we need to learn how to unleash our inner geniuses. As Dr. Treffert said in *Islands of Genius,* "The challenge is how to tap into those dormant abilities — the little Rain Man within us all — non-intrusively without some obtrusive central nervous system event. That's where the research is focused now."

Until the experts figure out how to do that, perhaps people could get a glimpse at the hidden nature of the universe through the sort of meditation practiced by Tibetan lamas or maybe someday by wearing a device like Dr. Snyder's creativity cap. It's exciting to think about other people getting to experience the world the way I do.

As I've settled into the new me, I've noticed that my life has started to turn around. I've been very fortunate this past year and have begun to share my work more. My art is getting noticed. I submitted work to a prestigious international art show called Art Basel for their Miami Beach event in 2008. My drawings were seen with the best contemporary artworks from around the world, and I won a Best International Newcomer award. Several art collectors have been in touch about acquiring my original drawings. Some of my work was just on display at Oxford University in England in an exhibit titled *Affecting Perception: Art & Neuroscience,* which featured artists with neurological conditions.

In the spring of 2012, *Nightline* did a report about me. I met journalist Neal Karlinsky and shared my view of the world as we walked through my favorite hometown park and visited Tacoma's Museum of Glass together. I never expected the world to light up the way it did after the report aired. The video and story went viral. There were thousands of Tweets, some by very prominent people. Could they really be interested in me? I wondered. Next, filmmakers and television producers were on the phone looking for me. One hilarious comedic television pitch had an actor portraying me working at Planet Futon while everyone in the world came to ask me for help, from schoolchildren with homework problems to NASA and the FBI. And then a woman sent me a photo: she'd gotten my double-slit experiment drawing tattooed on her right shoulder!

As a result of all this recent good fortune, I sign about ten autographs a week in the store. I feel a little embarrassed when people ask for my signature, but I see it as an opportunity to share more of my life and ask people about theirs. I make sure I spend time with each and every person, answering any questions he or she might have. People from all walks of life ask me things about the nature of the cosmos. Just recently a slim, blond woman of about forty came in with her husband to buy a futon for some overnight guests her family was having. We ended up spending four hours talking about relativity, parallel universes, pi, and all my favorite topics. I kept the store open two hours past closing time. It was so satisfying to me to share my ideas with receptive people.

Her mother came in the next day and said, "You've changed my daughter's life. She hasn't always been a happy person. She's had some bouts of depression. But she is so filled with wonder now and so energized. I've never seen her so alive. She said you explained things to her that were hidden to her before. She's looking at the world — and her place in it — a whole new way. Thank you." That touched me deeply.

Having so much to be grateful for has brought me to a place of acceptance and even forgiveness. If my attackers stood before me today, I would offer them an olive branch and express the hope that they've changed their lives for the better since that terrible night. I've come to the realization that if I carry around that hurt and anger forever, it will eat me alive, so I'm letting it go. You might say I've come full circle — and I've certainly felt every bump along the jaggy edge of the straight lines that I know make up one. I wonder if my assailants still carry the guilt and shame of what they did to me. It is my understanding they were never jailed, only arrested, held briefly, and then released.

I'm thankful that the epidemic of traumatic brain injuries is now finally coming into national awareness thanks to the research of a lot of top scientists and the work of victim advocates. I hope to be part of that growing national conversation.

One of the most notable recent developments came in early 2013 when Jorge Barrio, a professor of molecular and medical pharmacology, and a team of his fellow UCLA scientists released a small but groundbreaking study of five retired NFL players who each had a history of one or more concussions and who had some cognitive symptoms. The brain-imaging method Barrio developed allowed a marker of traumatic brain injury, a protein called tau, to be detected in living patients — previously, the only way to determine if this protein was present was at autopsy, when it was already too late to do anything about the findings. This new diagnostic is so important and such a huge breakthrough because early detection of damage may allow for some form of treatment and possibly even healing.

This explosive report grabbed headlines in the national media and boosted awareness of TBIs as a result. I felt a real kinship to those professional athletes and was happy to hear their stories being told. In fact, I was so moved that I decided to do all I could to advocate for TBI survivors. I would like to heed Dr. Treffert's call for me to be an ambassador for those who cannot speak about their injuries, especially the more than two hundred and fifty thousand U.S. servicemen and servicewomen who have suffered traumatic brain injuries since 2000.

I hope other TBI survivors can learn something from my journey, even if it is very rare, as Dr. Barrio said when he spoke to me and Maureen. In talking about his research and the relationship of my case to it, he said, "It's a very dramatic example of the things that could happen, how complex our brain is . . . Honestly, considering how devastating these concussions from beatings can be, I think it's a blessing that you can do all these things."

An extraordinary development in brain science occurred in early April 2013. That's when President Barack Obama made an announcement that really caught my attention. It was about something called the BRAIN Initiative, which stands for Brain Research through Advancing Innovative Neurotechnologies. I learned that a hundred million dollars was going to be dedicated to research on the human brain. In his speech, President Obama talked about giving scientists the tools and resources they needed to get a dynamic picture of the brain in action. That made me think of the fMRI tests I had undergone, and I wondered what new brain-imaging tests might be developed that could offer even better explanations of what is happening to me.

The program's creators hope to speed up the development of new technologies — kind of like how the space program produced huge technological side benefits. Getting better technology is only one goal of the project. Researchers will also be trying to gain a better understanding of how the brain works and how it is related to behavior and learning. With that comes a greater possibility of discovering new ways to treat or prevent disorders like Alzheimer's, autism, and even PTSD and traumatic brain injuries.

I already feel a personal connection with the BRAIN Initiative thanks to its co-chair William Newsome, a professor of neurobiology at Stanford University School of Medicine. Just one day after his appointment was announced, Dr. Newsome, who also serves as a board member of the Max Planck Institute for Biological Cybernetics and a correspondent for the committee on human rights at the National Academy of Sciences, took the time to comment thoughtfully on my story.

"Jason's case — and other cases like his, in which individuals develop new and specialized cognitive capabilities after brain injury — will be important sources of insight for us as we move forward with the BRAIN Initiative," he said. According to Dr. Newsome, people like me who suffer brain injuries and then undergo changes in behavior, perception, or personality can help brain scientists understand new things about the way the brain works. He pointed to new technologies on the horizon that may help scientists get an even clearer picture of what happens in the brains of people who suffer traumatic injuries and said that I might be extremely helpful. "Extraordinary clinical cases like Jason's, especially when examined using some of these new technologies, could give us insights into the brain that we would otherwise never have access to."

It's so exciting to think that my case might actually help scientists understand how the brain works and ultimately find better ways to diagnose and treat brain disorders. I would feel so honored if I could play a role — no matter how small — in improving the lives of TBI survivors, as well as the lives of sufferers of PTSD, chronic pain, depression, and OCD. And I love the idea that my experience and my brain may help boost awareness about the amazing gifts of synesthesia and savant syndrome.

What's even more thrilling is the very real possibility that with this new focus on brain research, scientists may finally find a way to unleash the inner genius hiding within each of us.

Since I began working on this book project, my wife, Elena, my daughter, Megan, and I have moved to a safer neighborhood in Tacoma. Living in a place that is not a hub of the criminal-justice system is such a relief and eases my mind tremendously as I plan my future. Elena graduated magna cum laude from the University of Washington and got a job at a major finance company. And my daughter, Megan, sixteen as of this writing, has blossomed into a beautiful young woman. She is learning Japanese and looking ahead to higher education. I take a special interest in her math studies and tutor her all I can. I'm so proud of them both and very lucky to have such a loving family. And our family is growing! Elena and I are expecting our first child together in August 2014.

I am now back in college part-time, taking classes at Highline Community College in my new neighborhood. I continue to try to synthesize what I believe due to my visions with what the accepted teachings are in these areas.

I still feel a lot of pressure to keep the family business going, but I have so many questions that can be answered only in an academic setting. I look forward to a lifetime of learning and remaining open, not hidden behind the walls of my home, despite any lingering fears and phobias. I hope to share my story with many more people in the coming years, demonstrating through my own experience that the extraordinary can happen in the lives of everyday people.

It's always just beneath the surface of us all.

Acknowledgments

T HIS BOOK MAY have two authors, but there are many team members behind its creation, without whom we'd still be talking between ourselves.

Our families and friends have been extremely supportive during this project — thank you especially to Elena and Megan Padgett and Dr. Erkan Ertürk, as well as Richard and Mary Seaberg, for listening and cheering and giving us the space to create.

To our literary agent, the immensely talented Stephen Barr: You started as our trusted compass and became our true north. Thank you for your early belief in this story (and that initial "Holy cow!"), for encouraging scenes where there were once mere sentences, and for your unfailing support throughout the publishing process. We realized early on there was more than one genius on this team.

To Dan Conaway and everyone at Writers House who also believed from the beginning and helped in so many ways: sincere thanks.

To our editor, the brilliant Courtney Young: You not only chose this story but elevated it with your high professional standards, elegant ideas, and sharp vision and focus. Thank you for such clarity and inspiration.

To everyone at Houghton Mifflin Harcourt, especially Naomi Gibbs and Beth Burleigh Fuller: We are so grateful for the help and investment from the start. To our copyeditor, the amazing and congenial Tracy Roe: You made everything more beautiful. We thank you for teaching us so much.

To Amanda and Dr. Paolo Padoan, Lynn Goode, Deborah Peterson, Dr. William C. Bushell, Dr. Neil Theise, Dr. William Lee, and Siobhan O'Leary—many thanks for reading and friendship and wisdom along the way.

Bibliography

Banissy, M. J., and J. Ward. "Mirror-Touch Synesthesia Is Linked with Empathy." *Nature Neuroscience* 10 (2007): 815–16. http://www.ncbi.nlm.nih.gov/pubmed/17572672.

Barnett, Kristine. *The Spark: A Mother's Story of Nurturing Genius.* New York: Random House, 2013.

Bartzokis, G., et al. "Lifespan Trajectory of Myelin Integrity and Maximum Motor Speed." *Neurobiology of Aging* 31 (2010): 1554–62. doi: 10.1016/j.neurobiolaging.2008.08.015.

Becker-Bense, S., et al. "Ventral and Dorsal Streams Processing Visual Motion Perception (FDG-PET Study)." *BMC Neuroscience* 13 (2012). doi: 10.1186/1471-2202-13-81.

Beckmann, Petr. *A History of Pi.* New York: St. Martin's Press, 1976.

Bialek, W. "Physical Limits to Sensation and Perception." *Annual Review of Biophysics and Biophysical Chemistry* 16 (1987): 455–78.

Bombardier, C. H., et al. "Rates of Major Depressive Disorder and Clinical Outcomes Following Traumatic Brain Injury." *Journal of the American Medical Association* 303 (2010): 1938–45. doi: 10.1001/jama.2010.599.

Brogaard, Berit, Simo Vanni, and Juha Silvanto. "Seeing Mathematics: Perceptual Experience and Brain Activity in Acquired Synesthesia." *Neurocase* (2012). doi: 10.1080/13554794.2012.701646.

Bushell, William C. "New Beginnings: Evidence That the Meditational Regimen Can Lead to Optimization of Perception, Attention, Cognition, and Other Functions." *Annals of the New York Academy of Sciences* 1172 (2009): 348–61.

Carvajal, D. "In Andalusia, on the Trail of Inherited Memories." *New York Times*, August 17, 2012. http://www.nytimes.com/2012/08/21/science/in-andalusia-searching-for-inherited-memories.html?pagewanted=all.

Cytowic, Richard. *The Man Who Tasted Shapes*. New York: Putnam, 1993.

———. "Synesthesia: Phenomenology and Neuropsychology: A Review of Current Knowledge." *Psyche* 2 (July 1995).

———. *Synesthesia: A Union of the Senses*. Cambridge, MA: Bradford, 2002.

Cytowic, Richard, and David Eagleman. *Wednesday Is Indigo Blue: Discovering the Brain of Synesthesia*. Cambridge, MA: MIT Press, 2011.

Dehaene, S., et al. "Cerebral Activations During Number Multiplication and Comparison: A PET Study." *Neuropsychologia* 34 (1996): 1097–1106.

Drew, L. B., and W. E. Drew. "The Contrecoup-Coup Phenomenon: A New Understanding of the Mechanism of Closed Head Injury." *Neurocritical Care* 1 (2004): 385–90. http://www.ncbi.nlm.nih.gov/pmc/articles/PMC3182015/.

Duffy, Patricia Lynne. *Blue Cats and Chartreuse Kittens: How Synesthetes Color Their Worlds*. New York: W. H. Freeman, 2001.

Feynman, Richard. *What Do You Care What Other People Think?: Further Adventures of a Curious Character*. New York: W. W. Norton, 1998.

Fischer, H. "U.S. Military Casualty Statistics: Operation New Dawn, Operation Iraqi Freedom, and Operation Enduring Freedom." *Congressional Research Service*. February 5, 2013. http://www.fas.org/sgp/crs/natsec/RS22452.pdf.

Gorman, James. "Brain as Clear as Jell-O for Scientists to Explore." *New York Times*, April 10, 2103. http://www.nytimes.com/2013/04/11/science/brains-as-clear-as-jell-o-for-scientists-to-explore.html.

Grandin, Temple. *Thinking in Pictures: My Life with Autism*. New York: Vintage, 2006.

Grandin, Temple, and Richard Panek. *The Autistic Brain: Thinking Across the Spectrum*. Boston: Houghton Mifflin Harcourt, 2013.

He, B. J., et al. "The Role of Impaired Neuronal Communication in Neurological Disorders." *Current Opinion in Neurology* 20: 655–60. http://www.nil.wustl.edu/labs/corbetta/PDFs%20for%20Web/The%20role%20of%20impaired%20neuronal%20communication%20in%20neurological%20disorders.pdf.

Krueger, F., et al. "Integral Calculus Problem Solving: An fMRI Investigation." *Neuroreport* 19 (2008): 1095–99.

Luminet, Jean-Pierre. "Science, Art and Geometrical Imagination." *Proceedings of the International Astronomical Union* 5 (January 2009): 248–73.

Luria, Alexander R., and Lynn Solotaroff. *The Mind of a Mnemonist: A Little Book about a Vast Memory.* Cambridge, MA: Harvard University Press, 1968.

Mandelbrot, Benoit B. "Fractal Geometry: What Is It, and What Does It Do?" *Proceedings of the Royal Society of London* 423 (1989): 3–16.

Mass, Wendy. *A Mango-Shaped Space.* Boston: Little, Brown Books for Young Readers, 2005.

McAllister, T. "Neurobiological Consequences of Traumatic Brain Injury." *Dialogues in Clinical Neuroscience* 13 (2011): 287–300.

Mumford, David, Caroline Series, and David Wright. *Indra's Pearls: The Vision of Felix Klein.* Cambridge: Cambridge University Press, 2002.

Piore, A. "When Brain Damage Unlocks the Genius Within." *Popular Science* (March 2013). http://www.popsci.com/science/article/2013-02/when-brain-damage-unlocks-genius-within?single-page-view=true.

Ramachandran, V. S., and Sandra Blakeslee. *Phantoms in the Brain: Probing the Mysteries of the Human Mind.* New York: William Morrow, 1998.

Ramachandran, V. S., and E. M. Hubbard. "Hearing Colors, Tasting Shapes." *Scientific American* (May 2003): 52–59.

Ramachandran, V. S., E. M. Hubbard, and P. A. Butcher. "'Higher' and 'Lower' Forms of Synesthesia May Arise from Cross-Wiring at Different Cortical Stages." *Journal of Vision* 2 (2002): 265. doi: 10.1167/2.7.265.

Rieke, F., and D. A. Baylor. "Single-Photon Detection by Rod Cells of the Retina." *Reviews of Modern Physics* 70 (1998): 1027–36.

Robinson, Sean. "Ten Years Later: Looking Back at Former Police Chief David Brame." *Tacoma News Tribune,* April 21, 2013.

Sacks, Oliver. *Musicophilia: Tales of Music and the Brain.* New York: Vintage Books, 2007.

———. "A Neurologist's Notebook: A Bolt from the Blue." *New Yorker,* July 23, 2007. http://www.newyorker.com/reporting/2007/07/23/070723fa_fact_sacks.

Seaberg, Maureen. *Tasting the Universe: People Who See Colors in Words and Rainbows in Symphonies.* New York: New Page Books, 2011.

Seghier, M. L. "The Angular Gyrus: Multiple Functions and Multiple Subdivisions." *Neuroscientist* 19 (2013): 43–61. doi: 10.1177/1073858412440596.

Small, G. W., et al. "PET Scanning of Brain Tau in Retired National Football League Players: Preliminary Findings." *Journal of the American Geriatrics Society* 21 (2012): 138–44. doi: 10.1016/j.jagp.2012.11.019.

Snyder, Allan. "Explaining and Inducing Savant Skills: Privileged Access to

Lower Level, Less-Processed Information." *Philosophical Transactions of the Royal Society* 364 (2009): 1399–1405.

Snyder, A. W., et al. "Savant-Like Skills Exposed in Normal People by Suppressing the Left Fronto-Temporal Lobe." *Journal of Integrative Neuroscience* 2 (2003): 149–58.

Stoica, B. A., and A. I. Faden. "Cell Death Mechanisms and Modulation in Traumatic Brain Injury." *Neurotherapeutics* 7 (2010): 3–12. doi: 10.1016/j.nurt.2009.10.023.

Tammet, Daniel. *Born on a Blue Day: Inside the Extraordinary Mind of an Autistic Savant*. New York: Free Press, 2007.

———. *Embracing the Wide Sky: A Tour Across the Horizons of the Mind*. New York: Atria Books, 2009.

———. *Thinking in Numbers: Of Life, Love, Meaning, and Math*. Boston: Little, Brown, 2013.

Taylor, Jill Bolte. *My Stroke of Insight: A Brain Scientist's Personal Journey*. New York: Plume, 2009.

Theise, Neil D., and M. C. Kafatos. "Complementarity in Biological Systems: A Complexity View." *Complexity* 18 (July/August 2013): 11–20.

———. "Sentience Everywhere: Complexity Theory, Panpsychism, and the Role of Sentience in Self-Organization of the Universe." *Journal of Consciousness, Exploration, and Research* 4 (April 2013): 378–90.

Treffert, Darold A. *Extraordinary People: Understanding Savant Syndrome*. New York: Ballantine Books, 1989.

———. *Islands of Genius: The Bountiful Mind of the Autistic, Acquired, and Sudden Savant*. London: Jessica Kingsley Publishers, 2010.

———. "The Savant Syndrome: An Extraordinary Condition. A Synopsis: Past, Present, Future." *Philosophical Transactions of the Royal Society* 364 (2009): 1351–57. doi: 10.1098/rstb.2008.0326.

Twomey, Steve. "Phineas Gage: Neuroscience's Most Famous Patient." *Smithsonian* (January 2010). http://www.smithsonianmag.com/history-archaeology/Phineas-Gage-Neurosciences-Most-Famous-Patient.html.

Van Campen, Cretien. *The Hidden Sense: Synesthesia in Art and Science*. Cambridge, MA: MIT Press, 2010.

Ward, Jamie. *The Frog Who Croaked Blue: Synesthesia and the Mixing of the Senses*. New York: Routledge, 2008.

Yomogida, Y., et al. "Mental Visual Synthesis Is Originated in the Fronto-Temporal Network of the Left Hemisphere." *Cerebral Cortex* 14 (2004): 1376–83.

Index